W9-COZ-722

# Always
# On Call

# ALWAYS ON CALL

When Illness

Turns Families

into Caregivers

*Edited by Carol Levine*

**Updated and Expanded Edition**

A United Hospital Fund Book

Vanderbilt University Press

NASHVILLE

This book is printed on acid-free paper.
Manufactured in the United States of America

*Library of Congress Cataloging-in-Publication Data*

Always on call : when illness turns families into
caregivers / edited by Carol Levine.
—2nd, updated and expanded ed.
    p. ; cm.
    "A United Hospital Fund Book."
    Includes bibliographical references and index.
ISBN 0-8265-1460-X (cloth : alk. paper)
ISBN 0-8265-1461-8 (pbk. : alk. paper)
    1. Caregivers. [DNLM: 1. Caregivers. 2. Home
Nursing. 3. Family. WY 200 A477 2004] I. Levine,
Carol. II. United Hospital Fund of New York.
RA645.3.A457 2004
362.1'4—dc22
                                    2004017369

# Contents

PART II

*The Impact of Caregiving*

# PART III

## *Responding to Caregivers' Needs*

# PART IV

## *Resources*

# Foreword

There are more than 27 million family caregivers in the United States—individuals who provide ongoing care to seriously ill or disabled family members. On the one hand, this figure reflects tremendous medical and technological progress. Medical advances in the last several decades are allowing patients to live longer with conditions that they would have died from in previous years. The explosion in home care technology permits seriously ill and disabled patients to remain in their homes much longer, rather than having to be routinely institutionalized to receive the care they need.

On the other hand, this figure reflects an extraordinary and growing amount of responsibility that is being placed on unpaid, largely untrained family members, who receive little support from the health care system in their efforts. Even a decade ago, much of the care that families must now assume was the province of paid clinicians in hospitals. A United Hospital Fund study found that the economic value of the care families provide at home amounts to more than home care and nursing home care costs combined. While family members often lovingly take on these care responsibilities, the personal and financial toll for doing so is mounting.

For the last several years, the United Hospital Fund, a health services research and philanthropic organization founded in 1879, has sought ways to ease these growing burdens on family caregivers. As part of its mission to shape positive change in health care in New York, it established the Families and Health Care Project in 1996, directed by Carol Levine, editor of this book. The project extends beyond the Fund's usual geographic focus to identify, on a national level, family caregivers' needs and ways that the health care system can better meet them. While a relatively modest undertaking, its $2 million grant-making initiative, which spurred the development of model programs by New York City health care institutions to provide greater support to caregivers, was the first of its kind in the country. Carol Levine's cutting-edge research and extensive efforts to raise public awareness about family caregiving have made major contributions to the national discussion about caregiving in both health care policy and delivery.

By capturing the new world of family caregiving in all its complexity and difficulty, this second edition of *Always On Call* takes this discussion to a critical new level. The extraordinary contributions of 22 authors—caregivers, caregiving advocates, and health care professionals—articulate the myriad, fundamental challenges that family caregivers face. For health care professionals and caregivers alike, *Always On Call* recognizes the vast contributions caregivers make, exposes the startling gaps in caregiver support services, and raises the bar on professional and societal responsibility to help. We hope that it inspires positive change in health care services and policy that will make family caregiving a more manageable, supported, and sustainable endeavor.

JAMES R. TALLON, JR.
President
United Hospital Fund

# Preface and Acknowledgments

The first edition of this book originated in a 1998 conference on family caregiving organized by the United Hospital Fund's Families and Health Care Project. At that time new research on the economic value of family caregiving and the findings of a series of United Hospital Fund focus groups of caregivers were presented for the first time. Since then, that information has been published in journals or United Hospital Fund reports.

Some of the most gripping moments of that day, however, would not have been captured for wider audiences without this book. Publishing the narratives of family caregivers and some of the workshop discussions was the impetus for the book; but the book quickly took on a momentum of its own. It soon grew to include more narratives and cover more issues than the conference that had inspired it.

The popularity of the first edition, and the rapidly advancing knowledge and experience in the field, led to a collaboration between the Fund and Vanderbilt University Press to publish this expanded and updated edition. This edition contains two new caregiver narratives, and updates by two of the caregivers whose narratives appeared in the first edition. Other chapters have been updated to incorporate new research and policy initiatives. A completely new section has been added with four chapters that address areas not covered in the first edition. Finally, the resource guide has been updated.

Many United Hospital Fund staff contributed advice, ideas, and information as this edition was created: David Gould, Deborah Halper, Sally Rogers, Phyllis Brooks, and Andrea Hart were good critics at every stage. Andrea Lucas, the Fund's editor, brought clarity and precision to every chapter. Michael Ames of the Vanderbilt University Press was an enthusiastic and supportive publisher throughout the process.

All the authors have our sincere thanks for their contributions. A special acknowledgment, however, goes to the family caregivers who revealed their most private and painful moments and feelings to convey the lived experience of caregiving. This book is immeasurably richer for their courage and their candor.

C.L.

# 1 Introduction: The Many Worlds of Family Caregivers

*Carol Levine*

Meet Marjorie, who could be your friend, neighbor, sibling, client, or you yourself. (She is fictional, so she could also be Mark.) She has been worried about her mother's failing memory for some time; now Florence, her mother, has broken her hip after falling in the bathroom. Florence has had successful surgery and is coming home from the hospital. She needs considerable assistance with her exercises, with medications and special diets for her pre-existing diabetes and heart disease, and with money management and household chores. Marjorie has already been helping out quite a lot, but her mother's level of need has increased dramatically. And it will go on increasing because, after all, Florence is 88, and being in the hospital seems to have made her more anxious and fearful.

The home care agency that is providing a few weeks of post-surgical care considers Marjorie the "responsible party," meaning that she will have to take charge if the home care aide does not show up or some other problem occurs. Researchers and policy makers consider Marjorie an "informal caregiver," because she is unpaid, although she is expected to perform the same tasks as a professional nurse and physical therapist. Secretaries and clerks at the various offices and agencies involved in Florence's care consider Marjorie "the daughter," that is, her mother's agent in providing documentation, arranging payment, and making and keeping appointments.

The other people in Marjorie's life have also responded to her pre-occupation with her mother. Marjorie's husband thinks she is spending too much time with her mother and too little with him and their three children, one of whom is a teenager going through difficult times. He doesn't like to bring it up, but Marjorie is also spending a lot of money for items her mother needs that are not covered by Medicare. Marjorie's employer is sympathetic but concerned because she takes so much time off from work and seems distracted even when she is on the job. Marjorie's friends tell her she is a "saint," but among themselves comment on how tired she looks and how she never seems to have time for lunch or a movie or even a phone call. Marjorie and Florence belong to the same church, and the minister comes to pray with Florence. He tells her how blessed she is to have such a good daughter, but he never asks Marjorie how she is coping with all the added responsibilities.

And what of Marjorie herself? She hardly has time to think about it, but she wants to be everything to everyone—a dutiful daughter, a loving wife and mother, a valued employee, and a good friend. She also has her own private interests and projects. Yet the role she has taken on with love, but without realizing the consequences to herself or others, does not easily allow for all her competing responsibilities.

Marjorie is a "family caregiver," a person who provides essential, unpaid assistance to a relative or friend who is ill, elderly, or disabled. The two parts of the term are equally important. "Family" denotes a special personal relationship with the care recipient, one based on birth, adoption, marriage, or declared commitment (Levine 1991). "Caregiver" describes the job, which may include providing personal care, carrying out medical procedures, managing a household, and interacting with the formal health care and social service systems on another's behalf. Caregivers are more than the sum of their responsibilities; they are real people with complex and often conflicted responses to the situations they face.

In the past few years, family caregiving has moved onto the health policy and professional practice agendas in new and urgent ways. This book is about family caregivers and also about health care and social service professionals and how they can provide much-needed assistance, advocacy, and advice.

## Family Caregivers in Context

As the narratives in the following chapters poignantly demonstrate, family caregivers may feel isolated, but they do not exist in isolation. Although typically considered part of the private realm of intimate relationships, family caregiving is greatly influenced by the cultural, political, and economic contexts of American society, all of which are dramatically changing families themselves. While family is a basic organizing structure of all human societies, definitions of family have varied throughout history and by culture. American society today is made up of many different types of families—multigenerational, biracial, nuclear, blended, adoptive, gay and lesbian partners and their children, and others.

Equally dramatic are the changes in U.S. demographics and health care. Although in earlier eras some individuals lived to great old age, the average life expectancy was decades less than it is now. Since 1900 the proportion of Americans aged 65 and older has more than tripled, from 4.1 percent to 12.4 percent in 2000 (U.S. Census Bureau 2001). In absolute terms, the number has increased from 3.1 million to 35 million. And the oldest of the old are increasing at an even higher rate. In the 1990s the most rapid growth, 38 percent, occurred among the very oldest—those 85 years and up—although this group still accounted for just 12 percent of the total population age 65 and up. More than half of older Americans, 53 percent, were between ages 65 and 74; 35 percent were 75 to 84 years old. Although the aging of the population is a national phenomenon, the number of older people, and thus of caregivers, varies from state to state. Some states are also more clearly affected than others by older adults' comprising larger proportions of their populations, beyond absolute numbers. Of the ten U.S. cities with populations of 100,000 or more and the greatest proportion of their residents 65 and older, for example, six are in Florida.

Old age does not necessarily equate with frailty or illness, but it does certainly bring with it an increase in diseases of aging, especially Alzheimer's; the older one gets, the more likely one is to have chronic illnesses or disabilities such as congestive heart failure, severe arthritis, or the sequelae of stroke. In the past, "nature" limited the need for caregiving; until the age of antibiotics, most people who suffered severe trauma or serious illness either got better on their own or died. But in the twentieth century, the advent of scientific medicine and the benefits of research, public health measures, and better nutrition and safer jobs enhanced and extended lives. Recent successes of acute care medicine—in the care of newborns and trauma patients, for example—have also created a population of adults dependent to unprecedented degrees on technology and on other people for basic survival.

Those other people are most often expected to be family members. But even in cultures where family is the primary unit of attachment, communities have usually supplemented what families can provide, or assumed some caregiving roles, such as helping new mothers or caring for the dying. Religious institutions have a long history of providing care for the ill and dying; modern hospitals grew out of this tradition. Until the 1970s and 1980s, in the United States people who were ill frequently stayed in hospitals for weeks and months "convalescing." Relatives with psychiatric problems, mental retardation, severe disabilities, and other conditions were routinely institutionalized on physicians' advice. The shortcomings of care and abuses of human rights that were uncovered, as well as the economic costs, are powerful deterrents, however, to a return to institutionalization for these populations.

Yet present-day realities create a tension between the poles of family-centered and professional care; old assumptions and patterns of care no longer hold. While the prevalence of chronic rather than acute illness would argue for home care, women's increasing participation in the labor market makes the role of stay-at-home caretaker less tenable than ever. Overriding that limitation, however, and probably most decisive of all, is the ongoing push toward a health care delivery and financing system that uses hospitals and professional and public resources sparingly and patients' homes and family caregivers liberally.

The process of market-driven health care is still evolving, but trends are clear. Health care costs are being contained through reduced length of hospital stays, increased outpatient and community-based care, and reductions in home care benefits available through insurance, managed care organizations, or public programs. Individuals and families are under increased pressure to pay more direct costs. At the same time, with the emergence of industries marketing high-tech medical equipment for home use, families are expected to provide ever more hands-on, often technologically complex, care.

Most families do not want and cannot afford to place their loved ones in long-term care facilities; only 4.5 percent of Americans over 65 live in nursing homes, a decline from 5.1 percent in 1990. While alternatives such as assisted living have grown in the past decade, they are generally too expensive for most families. These economic and technological developments mean that family caregivers are being asked to shoulder greater burdens for longer periods of time, and to forgo more educational, career, and social opportunities for themselves. Indeed, the human and social costs of maintaining patients at home are very high.

## Economic Value of Family Caregivers' Work

Clearly, family caregivers provide a substantial amount of free labor that undergirds the entire health care system. Nevertheless, until 1999 this vital aspect of the trillion-dollar U.S. health care economy had not been calculated in economic terms. What would the economic value of this care be, if it were treated as employment in the health care marketplace? A study commissioned by the United Hospital Fund's Families and Health Care Project addressed this question, using three sets of values to produce high, midrange, and low estimates (Arno, Levine, and Memmott 1999). Based on large national data sets, the midrange estimate for the number of caregivers in 1997 was 25.8 million. The number of hours, on average, provided per week by each caregiver was held constant at 17.9, the only national figure then available. Using a midrange wage of $8.18/hour, the authors estimated that the midrange national economic value of informal caregiving in 1997 was $196 billion; that number had increased to $257 billion by 2000, based on 27.3 million caregivers averaging more than 20 hours of care per week at a midrange wage of $8.81/hour, as shown in Figure 1 (Arno 2002). This figure dwarfs that year's national expenditures for both formal home health care, $32 billion, and nursing home care, $92 billion. This estimate of the economic value of informal caregiving is equivalent to approximately 20 percent of total national health care expenditures of $1.3 trillion (Figure 2).

By revealing family caregiving to be an integral and critically large component of the health care system, the study took the issue from the micro level of individuals attempting to cope with the stresses and responsibilities of caregiving to the macro level of a system in part depen-

## Figure 1. Economic Value of Informal Caregiving, U.S., 2000

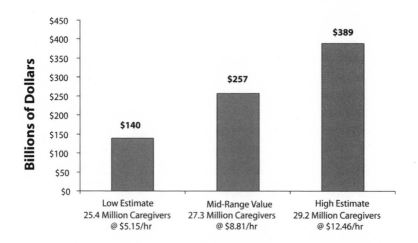

Source: Arno, PS. 2002. Economic value of informal caregiving. Paper presented at the meeting of the American Association for Geriatric Psychiatry, Orlando, FL.

dent on those individuals. Clearly the health care system must find more effective and meaningful ways to support and sustain family caregivers.

### Giving Family Caregivers a Voice

Formal studies of family caregivers of sick and elderly people proliferated in the 1970s and 1980s. Stimulated by the establishment of Medicare and Medicaid and the expenditure of public funds on medical care, many of these studies focused on program beneficiaries and their caregivers. Other studies looked at seriously ill people with specific diseases, especially Alzheimer's, to characterize the stress and burden on their caregivers. Although the resulting literature provided much valuable information, most of the data were gathered in an era when health care costs were increasing rapidly, government programs were expanding, and the impact of advanced home care technology had yet to be felt. Managed care was still a gleam in a few cost-conscious economists' eyes.

To gain a richer understanding of caregiving, the United Hospital Fund (the Fund) and the Visiting Nurse Service of New York (VNS) collaborated with the Harvard University School of Public Health on a national, population-based survey of family caregivers. The survey, "Long-Term Care

**Figure 2. Home Care, Nursing Home Care, Informal Caregiving, and National Health Expenditures, U.S., 2000**

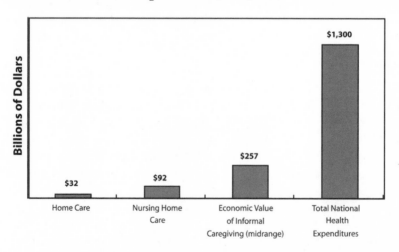

Expenditure data from HCFA, Office of the Actuary, Levit K et al. 2002. *Health Affairs* 21.
Source: Arno PS. 2002. Economic value of informal caregiving. Paper presented at the meeting of the American Association for Geriatric Psychiatry, Orlando, FL.

from the Caregiver's Perspective," was conducted by the National Opinion Research Center (NORC) at the University of Chicago, with funding from the Henry J. Kaiser Family Foundation (Donelan et al. 2002). The Fund and the VNS also funded an over-sample of New York City respondents, permitting an analysis of the city's specific experience as well. Interestingly, the New York City data do not differ in critical ways from the national results (Levine et al. 2000). For both parts of the study, valuable benchmark data were drawn from a national survey of 1,509 caregivers conducted in 1996, using similar methodology (National Alliance for Caregiving and the American Association of Retired Persons [NAC/AARP] 1997).

The survey elicited information about several important but little-studied issues, especially probing caregivers' relationships with the formal medical care system. Guided by earlier research conducted by the Fund (Levine 1998), the survey attempted to learn more about the transition from hospital to home care. Because the hospital discharge process is too often hurried and incomplete, the survey asked family caregivers whether they received any training to prepare them to perform complex medical tasks and assist with personal care "activities of daily living" (ADLs); what any such training covered; and who provided it. But with the full caregiving experience going well beyond the hospital-to-home transition—for many family members it is a long-term commitment—caregivers were also asked about their interactions over time with staff of the formal health care system, including home care nurses and home health aides. Additionally, the survey tried to explore caregivers' perceptions of needs that were not met by the formal care system, and their understanding of why those needs remained unmet.

The survey deliberately defined "caregiver" broadly, as anybody who provides unpaid help or arranges for paid or unpaid help for a relative or friend who is unable to do some things for him- or herself because of illness, disability, or age. The help given could be with personal care or medical needs, or with "instrumental activities of daily living" (IADLs) such as household chores, logistical tasks, or finances; the person receiving help could be living in the caregiver's home, in his/her own home, or in another place such as a nursing home.

This definition covers a wide range of relationships and tasks, both those traditionally associated with caregiving and less traditional activities such as arranging or paying for care. Of 4,874 respondents who completed a screening interview in early 1998, survey researchers identified 1,002 caregivers for the national sample; 402 additional caregivers were interviewed for the New York City sample. Interviews were conducted in either English or Spanish. The sample was weighted to reflect the general population, which affects the sample size throughout the report.[1]

## The Parameters of Caregiving

Roughly one in five persons (21.8 percent) reported that they were current caregivers or had cared for someone within the previous 12 months. Who are these people, and whom are they assisting? What is it that they're doing, and how big a job is it? The survey produced a wealth of detailed information from both the national and New York perspectives, as noted earlier (Donelan et al. 2002; Levine et al. 2000). Key points among those findings follow here:[2]

- Caregiving is usually assumed to be, and in many respects remains, "women's work." Nevertheless, this population-based survey identified many more male caregivers than had previous surveys of specific groups of caregivers. While surveys have typically found women outnumbering men by three to one (NAC/AARP 1997), we found that 53.7 percent of caregivers were female and 46.3 percent were male. Caregivers were also younger than expected. Almost equal proportions were between the ages of 18 and 39 years (42.7 percent) and 40 and 64 years (43.9 percent). Not surprisingly, then, more than half (52.6 percent) were employed full-time. Over half the sample (60 percent) was married.

   Most care recipients were female (65.3 percent). Almost two-thirds were older than 64, and almost half of that group were 80 years or older. Nevertheless, it is important to remember that young and middle-aged adults constitute a large segment of persons receiving care: 28 percent of care recipients were between the ages of 19 and 64 years, and 6.7 percent were chronically ill or disabled children under 18.

   Care recipients were most often (41.8 percent) a parent of their caregiver; another third were grandparents, aunts, uncles, cousins, siblings, or other relatives. Only 6.8 percent of care recipients were spouses, and 1 percent companions or partners—most likely because many elderly women had never married or had outlived their spouses or partners.

   Over a third of care recipients (37 percent) lived alone. Caregivers and care recipients shared a residence in 28.8 percent of cases; another 21.8 percent of care recipients lived in the home of another family member or friend. Relatively few lived in nursing homes or other group living situations (7.8 percent and 4.6 percent respectively).

- The great majority of care recipients (73.9 percent) had one or more serious health problems, caregivers reported, including heart disease, osteoarthritis, diabetes, and/or cancer. Roughly one in ten had Alzheimer's, senility, dementia, or other cognitive impairment. Many caregivers, however, could give only a vague description of care recipients' health problems, or attributed those problems to "old age." This finding suggests that some health care professionals are not communicating adequately with caregivers about their patient's diagnosis and, by inference, prognosis and treatment. Significantly, 54.6 percent of care recipients had been hospitalized in the past year. Also significant: caregivers, as a group, are in vulnerable health as well, with nearly a third (32.3 percent) reporting serious health problems of their own.

- Over half those surveyed (51.1 percent) reported that they were the primary caregiver, the one who, aside from paid help, "provides/provided most care." Their reasons varied from the pragmatic—58.2 percent lived closest to the care recipient, and 43.2 percent were the family members with the most time—to the diplomatic, with more than a third (37.1 percent) reporting that the care recipient did not want strangers in the home. Four in ten caregivers (39.8 percent) cited care recipients' inability to afford paid help. Many (43.8 percent) reported that care recipients did not require professional help—although it was not clear whether a health professional, the caregiver, or the care recipient had made that judgment. Only one in eight (12.2 percent) said the care recipient had been discharged from the hospital too soon.

- Some caregivers spent a lot of time and energy fulfilling their responsibilities; for others, the tasks were less time-consuming and intense. On average, caregivers spent an estimated 20.9 hours per week providing care, more time than the 1997 NAC/AARP estimate of an average of 17.9 hours per week. Six in ten caregivers reported spending less than 20 hours a week, with some providing "episodic" care of only an hour a week, but 17 percent provided "constant" care of 60 or more hours per week.

    Although, as noted earlier, we found that more men were caregivers than had been expected, we also learned how different their roles were from women's. Men provided neither as much care, measured in hours per week, nor as intensive care, as gauged by the study's measure of intensity, described later. Nearly two-thirds of the male caregivers provided less than 20 hours of care per week, and only 10.5 percent put in 60 or more hours per week. Among female respondents, more than half (54.9 percent) also provided fewer than 20 hours per week of care, but nearly 23 percent provided 60 or more hours per week.

For most of those surveyed, caregiving was of long duration. Four in ten (40.8 percent) reported that they had been caregivers for five or more years. Over a third (37.3 percent) had been caregiving for one to four years, and only 21.9 percent had been caregivers for less than one year.

• Use of the Level of Care Index that was included in the NAC/AARP study—measuring the intensity of caregiving, on a scale of one (least intensive) to five (most)—revealed a roughly bell-shaped distribution (Levine et al. 2000). Approximately 40 percent of all caregivers provided the two lowest levels of care, and a nearly identical proportion provided the two highest levels. While the experience of caregiving is not driven by a large number of people providing small amounts of service, neither are all caregivers consumed by their tasks.

• Caregiver tasks ranged from ADLs and IADLs to medically related activities. Over 25 percent of caregivers performed each ADL, or personal care task, except managing incontinence (17.2 percent) and feeding (16.7 percent). More than half the caregivers provided assistance with each IADL except financial tasks (and nearly half the respondents handled those) and arranging for government assistance programs such as Medicare or Medicaid. The highest proportion of caregivers performed shopping or errands (84.8 percent), drove or helped care recipients with public transportation (75.6 percent), and did housework (71.1 percent).

But many caregivers are doing far more than personal care and household tasks. Significantly, the survey found caregivers deeply involved in medically related tasks. More than a third (39.1 percent) provided help with prescription medications, given orally, by injection, intravenously, by infusion pump, or by suppository. Almost a fifth (19.1 percent) changed dressings or bandages, and 14.7 percent helped with equipment such as oxygen, home dialysis, tubes, or catheters.

- As anticipated, the survey found that recent hospitalization had a major impact on the kind of care provided. And it is critically important to remember that 54.6 percent of care recipients had been hospitalized within the past year. That population required more assistance in every category of ADLs than did care recipients who had not been hospitalized—so that their caregivers were more than half again as likely to bathe them or manage their incontinence, and more than twice as likely to help them with dressing, feeding, getting in and out of bed, and walking across the room.

  Hospitalization had somewhat less impact on IADLs, because most caregivers already performed a substantial number of these tasks, regardless of the health status of the care recipient. Those caring for a loved one who had been hospitalized were twice as likely to do shopping and one-and-a-half times as likely to make telephone calls on behalf of the care recipient as caregivers serving persons who had not been hospitalized in the past year.

  Likewise, caregivers of persons who had been hospitalized were nearly twice as likely to change dressings or bandages and almost three times as likely to be helping with medical equipment as those caring for persons who had not been hospitalized. Caregivers of recently hospitalized persons were only slightly more likely to help with prescription medications than those caring for persons who had not been hospitalized, which suggests the prevalence of medication use among a largely chronic-care population.

- The relationship between hospitalization and duration of care was complex. Interestingly, caregivers of recently hospitalized persons were only half as likely to have been providing care for an extended period—more than five years. Most probably hospitalization in the past year was the trigger that precipitated the need for home care, the source of which was likely the family.

  While recent hospitalization did not significantly influence the number of hours of care provided each week, it had a dramatic impact on the intensity of care. Caregivers for the recently hospitalized were twice as likely to be giving care at Level 4 or 5 of the intensity scale than those caring for persons who had not been recently hospitalized. This may explain why these caregivers were also almost twice as likely to hire or arrange for some type of formal home care, such as a nurse or home care aide.

- A disturbing proportion of caregivers reported receiving no instruction in the tasks of caregiving. More than half (56.9 percent) were taught nothing about ADLs, some of which require specific techniques and are considerably more difficult and involved when performed for an ill or disabled individual. Almost a third (31.4 percent) of those who changed dressings or bandages, for which technique is also clearly important, received no training. And just under a fifth of those who helped with medical equipment and of those who administered prescription medications reported receiving no instructions on those tasks (18.1 percent and 19 percent, respectively).

    Instruction, when it came, could issue from either the formal system (nurses, doctors, or other professionals to whom they made referrals) or from informal sources that caregivers themselves identified. The formal system was most effective in instructing people about medications and medical equipment, with nearly three-quarters of caregivers (72 percent and 69.8 percent respectively) citing some professional direction on these aspects of care. Far fewer respondents (58.7 percent) reported formal instruction on changing dressings and bandages. For each medical task, in fact, some caregivers had to turn to an informal source of help, typically a neighbor, a relative with a health care background, or some other acquaintance. Reliance on this type of non-system instruction injects an element of chance at best and of risk at worst.

    Caregivers employed full time were less likely than others to receive system-directed instruction—less than half as likely, in the case of dressing and bandage changes. That may be due to working caregivers' inability to be there when care recipients were discharged from the hospital, or at other opportunities for instruction.

- Among caregivers who performed ADLs, slightly more than a third (34.2 percent) reported feeling "not at all," "not very," or only "somewhat" comfortable—rather than "very comfortable"—about these tasks. Similarly, about a third of those performing medical tasks had some reservations about their competence—with 30.3 percent not feeling totally capable of managing dressings and bandages, and 35 percent concerned about their ability to help with medical equipment. A smaller but still high percentage (22.1 percent) said they felt less than completely capable of managing prescription medications.

Particularly instructive was the finding that those who spent 20 hours or more a week caregiving were twice as likely as those devoting less time to it to report that it was somewhat or very difficult: persons providing more care do not necessarily develop a greater sense of competence and self-assurance. And surveys that look only at tasks performed to measure burden may miss another important dimension: caregivers assess difficulty not just by tasks but by the whole experience. That includes relationships with the care recipient, other family members, and the formal care system, and the time and energy subtracted from the rest of the caregiver's life.

In fact, caregivers were more negative about the overall experience of caregiving than about specific tasks. In evaluating caregiving as an overall experience, more than 42 percent had issues with the process, with 33.8 percent saying it was "somewhat difficult" and 8.7 percent calling it "very difficult." Only 34.6 percent reported that caregiving was "not at all difficult" and 22.9 percent said it was "not very difficult."

- Only a small proportion of caregivers hired or arranged for additional help from one or more paid professionals, such as a nurse or physical therapist (17.7 percent), or paraprofessionals, such as a home care aide (9.4 percent).[3] Those caregivers who did bring in paid help were more than three times as likely as those who did not to be providing care at Levels 4 or 5 of the Care Index. Clearly, paid assistance did not release caregivers from their roles, but only supplemented their very considerable levels of service. Significant needs following a hospitalization may be the key factor contributing to this pattern.

  Caregivers' perceptions of the quality of formal assistance were mixed. The overwhelming majority of caregivers who had hired or arranged for paid help in the past year reported good to excellent care by both paid professionals (83 percent) and home care aides (82 percent). Yet a notable proportion of those caregivers also reported worrying about mistreatment or neglect of care recipients by both professionals (23.3 percent) and paraprofessionals (18.9 percent).

- Almost a fifth (17.9 percent) of survey respondents reported a need for help, in the previous year, that they were unable to obtain. More than half of that group (55.5 percent) reported unmet medical need (for a nurse, for instance), and 71.2 percent reported unmet non-medical need (e.g., for a home care aide). Caregivers attributed such unmet needs to:

-   Access-related difficulties (41.8 percent), including refusal of service by doctors or hospitals, problems with services or transportation, the lack of an available doctor or nurse, or a "government decision" that the care recipient did not need the services;
-   Financial difficulties (36.4 percent), including inability to pay for services, insurance problems, and ineligibility for government assistance, based on income or financial assets; and/or
-   Family problems (21.8 percent), including disagreements about who should provide care, not having enough time or strength, or caregiver illness.

The perception, then, is that obstacles to care in the main reflect some type of systemic problem, and are not the result of familial disagreements or inability to marshal caregiving resources.

## Differences in Family Capacity for Caregiving

The survey results and the other chapters in this book paint a picture of great variability among caregivers and care recipients, and failures of the health care and social service systems to meet their needs. How should professionals and policy makers respond? One of the major goals for the future should be to recognize and address appropriately the many kinds of diversity among family caregivers that are reflected in this book—diversity of family structures and relationships; sources of strength and stress; caregiving needs required for particular medical, behavioral, and social conditions; duration and intensity of caregiving; and availability of formal and informal resources, to name a few. Differences in family circumstances are crucial factors in determining the level and kind of family responsibility that is both fair and achievable. Some families cope very well in exceptionally trying situations with little or no outside assistance. Others find the burdens overwhelming: substandard home care, potential abuse and neglect, and eventual institutionalization of the family member, poor health for the caregiver, and sometimes irrevocable family dissension and impoverishment may result.

Current policies and programs are generally based on only rough assessments of these crucial differences. Discharge planning focuses on the immediate, short-term care plan, but what can be done for a few weeks or months may not be supportable for longer periods. The patient's status as Medicaid- or Medicare-eligible may be considered the only relevant factor in determining a plan, rather than a starting point for determining what additional needs must be met through other resources.

Indeed, caregiver and family capacity must be weighed along with patient need in proposing an appropriate plan. "Capacity" is shorthand for the many factors that affect a caregiver's and a family's ability to provide and sustain long-term home care. But while several assessment tools for measuring caregiver burden and stress are available, and others are in development, there is little focus on the family as a whole. A fully developed measure would more precisely rank and weigh the various factors that together determine capacity. For introductory purposes, however, it is assumed that a high, moderate, and low capacity can be assessed.

Among the tangible factors are the number of people available to provide care, family economic resources, home setting (whether the caregiver lives with the patient or not), distance of other family members from the patient's home, and other family responsibilities, such as small children and/or other ill or elderly members. Also important are such intangibles as family dynamics, whether the family is "individualistic" (members tend to maintain separate and independent lives while at the same time having loving relationships with their family members) or "collectivist" (members see the family as one unit, in which anything that affects one of them affects them all). Cultural and religious traditions are clearly significant. "Social support"—through formal membership in religious institutions, service organizations, or other groups, and informal relationships with congregation members or others—are also elements in the calculus.

Many families cannot be clearly defined as high, moderate, or low capacity. Some of their characteristics fit one category, but other features fall into another group. A family may, for example, have many available members but little ability to cooperate among themselves. Or they may have substantial financial resources but also many members with compelling medical, educational, or other needs. Situations in which there is a primary caregiver but little family or social support are probably among the most tenuous.

Patient needs include not only the strictly medical but also assistance with ADLs, paying bills and managing other financial matters, emotional support, and social services. Here, too, there may be inconsistencies. A patient with high needs in one area may have only moderate or low needs in another. Someone with a spinal cord injury, for example, may require considerable assistance with dressing and other activities of daily living but may be totally independent in managing financial matters and other intellectual activities. A person with a progressive disease that affects mental functioning, on the other hand, may require minimal physical assistance and extensive behavioral monitoring.

In some cases patient needs and family capacity coincide. A patient with multiple, extensive needs may be fortunate enough to have family members and friends who can meet all those demands without excessively draining their personal and familial reserves. Or a family with modest resources may be able to care quite adequately for a patient requiring relatively little assistance. But in most situations the match is not quite so perfect. Patients may need help of a kind and intensity that a family is hard put to provide. Family members may be devoted and caring but simply live too far away to provide ongoing daily care. Or they may be able to manage the nontechnical aspects of care but not a highly complicated medical regimen.

When family capacity cannot fulfill all patient needs, some services and supports will have to be supplied by outside sources. Some of what is required can be put in place by community or volunteer resources, and other elements by formal, professionally trained personnel. An accurate measure of capacity thus might help families and care planners arrive at agreement on what constitutes a reasonable set of services, as the following two examples illustrate.

Mr. A is a 77-year-old man whose first bout with colon cancer occurred ten years ago. In the past three years several recurrences, and new rounds of treatment, have left him increasingly dependent. Currently he is receiving intravenous chemotherapy at home, and requires frequent medical monitoring and adjustment of his medications. He is weak and needs assistance with bathing, toileting, feeding, and other ADLs. He can only eat specially prepared food. Although there is some hope that treatment will lead to remission, the oncologist is beginning to talk about palliative care and perhaps hospice. Mr. A has been married for forty years; he and his wife have a married daughter, a married son, and an unmarried son. Mr. A also has a sister and brother whose families have been very close to him. He is a prominent member of his church and has been active in several civic groups.

The whole family has discussed the division of labor at key points in the illness; though the tasks are not divided equally, there is family unity about what is needed and how it should be provided. Through his illness

Mr. A's wife and daughter have provided most of his care, with frequent help from the other children and his sister's family. The unmarried son, who has a thriving business in another city, has made significant financial contributions to offset the many medical costs not covered by Medicare or supplemental insurance.

Mr. A's family is understandably upset at their relative's evident decline. They need counseling about available options and dealing with his anticipated death. They also need home care visits by trained medical professionals and instruction in how to manage the care regimen and potential emergencies. They need someone they can call with questions. On the plus side, family members can relieve each other and provide needed respite; community members can help with food, shopping, chores, and emotional support as well. The family is going through a crisis that they need help in managing, but they have the necessary strength and resources to handle the challenge. Even with today's limited external resources, it is possible for the necessary supports to be put in place.

Now consider Mr. Z, whose medical condition echoes Mr. A's. With little assistance available from his family, and few contacts in the community, he is in desperate straits. His three children live in distant cities; one is in the armed forces, one has a severely handicapped child, and the third is struggling to overcome alcoholism. Only an elderly sister and a niece live nearby; neither speaks English fluently and both are easily intimidated by the bureaucratic systems they encounter in trying to obtain help. They do what they can, but are soon overwhelmed by the intensity of Mr. Z's needs. Physicians, nurses, and home health aides are needed to stabilize and monitor his condition. Counseling and support from the rest of their family and from friends and neighbors are needed to maintain the sister's and niece's commitment. A social worker is needed to coordinate all the services necessary to keep this patient at home, including hospice or palliative care as appropriate. In fact, Mr. Z may not be a candidate for home hospice because of the paucity of family resources to provide the bulk of care.

These scenarios only approximate the complexities of real cases and real families. Between Mr. A and Mr. Z there are, of course, myriad families who fall somewhere along the continuum of need. The enormous diversity of family capacities should be considered in developing appropriate care plans. Equally important is the need to re-evaluate these plans at regular intervals and with changes in the patient's condition, family circumstances, or other related factors.

Additionally, these scenarios don't address one of the most important questions of all: Who should pay for this care? It would be too simplistic, to say nothing of unrealistic, to assume that public programs should pick up all the unmet needs for family support, once they are identified. But it would be equally simplistic to assume that families can pay for all the services they need on their own. Some combination of enhanced private insurance benefits, the services of voluntary health organizations and community agencies where appropriate, and adequate public funds for serious circumstances could make a major difference. Coordination of existing services and communication among service providers as well as with patients and families would in itself be a significant benefit. Public as well as private funds can also be used for training professionals and paraprofessionals to recognize the special needs of family caregivers and to provide more effective services than now exist.

Private foundations can also play a role in supporting and evaluating innovative programs. The Family Caregiving Grant Initiative, a four-year, $2 million initiative supported by the United Hospital Fund, is an example (Levine 2003). Most interventions related to caregiving come in times of crisis, when fragile support systems fail and families can no longer cope. Planning at the outset that realistically assesses what families can do on their own and where they need support—and then fills the gap to the extent possible—should in the long run prove not only more compassionate but also more effective.

Throughout this book the authors illustrate the diversity of family caregivers' experiences and needs. They bring together both quantitative and qualitative data to present a well-rounded picture of family caregivers and to suggest ways to support them through programs, policies, and practices. Caregivers come from and live in many different worlds. The following chapters bring those worlds to life.

## Notes

1. In addition to this weighting of sample size, proportions and percentages may differ slightly from other published works on these data for various reasons, including alternative methods of coding, distinct definitions of variable categorization, use of missing data, and different methods of data cleaning. Despite these minor irregularities, the findings are consistent. For a more detailed description of methodologies, refer to Levine et al. 2000.
2. The following data appear in somewhat different form in Gould D. 2004. Family caregivers and the health care system: Findings from a national survey. In Levine C and TH Murray, eds. *The cultures of caregiving: Value conflicts and*

*common ground among families, professionals, and policy makers.* Baltimore: Johns Hopkins University Press.
3.  N=1,057. Due to the wording of the question, more people may have received formal care than the question captured. This finding is consistent, however, with other national studies, in which the vast majority of people received only "informal" care.

## References

Arno PS. 2002. Economic value of informal caregiving. Paper presented at the meeting of the American Association for Geriatric Psychiatry, Orlando, FL.

Arno PS, C Levine, and MM Memmott. 1999. The economic value of informal caregiving. *Health Affairs* 18(2): 182-8.

Donelan K, CA Hill, C Hoffman, K Scoles, PH Feldman, C Levine, and D Gould. 2002. Challenged to care: Informal caregivers in a changing health system. *Health Affairs (Millwood)* 21(4): 222-31.

Levine C. 1991. AIDS and changing concepts of family. In Nelkin D, DP Willis, and SV Parris, eds. *A disease of society: Cultural and institutional responses to AIDS.* Cambridge: Cambridge University Press.

———. 1998. *Rough crossings: Family caregivers' odysseys through the health care system.* New York: United Hospital Fund.

———. 2003. *Making room for family caregivers: Seven innovative hospital programs.* New York: United Hospital Fund.

Levine C, AN Kuerbis, D Gould, M Navaie-Waliser, PH Feldman, and K Donelan. 2000. *A survey of family caregivers in New York City: Findings and implications for the health care system.* New York: United Hospital Fund.

National Alliance for Caregiving and the American Association of Retired Persons. 1997. *Family caregiving in the U.S.: Findings from a national survey.* Bethesda, MD, and Washington, DC: National Alliance for Caregiving and AARP.

U.S. Census Bureau. 2001. *The 65 years and over population: 2000.* Washington, DC: U.S. Census Bureau, 1.

PART I

*Voices of
Family
Caregivers*

# 2

# First My Mother, Then My Aunt: A Caregiver's Diary of Alzheimer's Disease

*Carol Ann Young*

My mother was the third youngest of 11 children born to a woman who died from a fever when Mother was very young. My grandfather was a foundry worker who earned $19.00 a week making farm plows. He didn't marry again, so the older children raised the younger ones. They grew their own food, had a well, fruit trees, chickens, and pigs. Most of the siblings followed each other north to Harlem from Virginia. They came with thousands of other southern African Americans who were looking for job opportunities in the first few decades of the twentieth century. By 1990 there were five surviving sisters: my mother and the oldest in Harlem, the youngest in the Bronx, the next-to-the-youngest in Virginia, and an older sister in Washington, DC.

We gather for family celebrations, loss, and occasional visits. We're not frequent callers, but when we see a need, we are vigilant and devoted to each other. We are a committed extended family.

In 1983 I started a graphic design business out of my apartment. It's a difficult and highly competitive field, so my life became centered around my business. In 1985 my sister and I moved my mother into my apartment building. I was very busy and Mother, a private person, and I had little contact except for family gatherings.

## 1990: The First Signs

In 1990, Mother still lived alone: independent, proud, a retired New York City clerk, and widowed a dozen years. She was 77 years old, and my sister and I were becoming increasingly concerned about her behavior. She had become withdrawn, unusually secretive and fearful, and began avoiding other family members.

Mother began to experience difficulty going to the bathroom, and she reached out to us for help. I found a specialist, and my sister and I accompanied Mother to her appointments. We learned that her condition could be remedied with surgery. Mother was emotional, confused, anxious, suspicious, and unable to retrieve the words she needed to communicate effectively with the doctor. The strong, capable mother we knew was giving way to a helpless, childlike woman we had occasionally seen before, but not to this degree. We were used to a woman who kept her physical problems private and handled her own business. She said she didn't know what to do, so the three of us discussed the prospect of surgery. She asked me to take care of her medical bills and insurance forms.

In June she was bumped by a cab while trying to cross 34th Street. She was taken to St. Clare's Hospital and Health Center with a minor leg injury. In October her youngest sister died.

## 1991: My Aunt Reaches Out

In April 1991, Mother underwent the surgery. In October, my sister moved from her Bronx co-op to Colorado. Mother became more fearful, withdrawn, and anxious. She needed to be reminded of her follow-up appointments and escorted to the doctor's office.

My aunt, Mother's older sister, lived two blocks away. She was 83 years old, independent, proud, a retired nurse, active, never married, with no children. In April she had told me that her dentist recommended gum surgery to correct a fitting problem with her dentures. She didn't want to have surgery and didn't know what to do. I arranged for her to see another dentist and accompanied her to the appointments. It was the first time she had reached out to me for any kind of help. Normally, we didn't talk much, but I had been calling her to get advice about my mother's behavior.

## 1992: The Problems Escalate

By 1992, Mother needed a lot of attention, help, and care. She was calling frequently, demanding to visit while I was working, asking for assistance, or just wanting to talk. She was having difficulty counting her change and became suspicious of the cashiers at the grocery store. She suspected that someone was trying to get into her apartment because she was having problems operating her lock and keeping track of her keys. She had her lock changed. She became confused about the days, the time, the seasons. She was frustrated, anxious, and walking unsteadily. She insisted that I help her do the things she was having difficulty with instead of letting me do them for her, so I began to routinely escort her to the bank, the grocery store, and the doctor. She was desperately trying to maintain her independence. She attended my nephew's June wedding in Florida. From there she went to Colorado with my sister. In August she asked me to change her lock again.

I was alarmed by how much time her care was absorbing. The paperwork and follow-up required by her Medicare and other insurance forms were extensive. Business was slow, and I needed to pay serious attention to earning a living and pursuing new clients. Besides the new tasks, her care was becoming emotionally exhausting. I worried about her. She was excessively manipulative with blame and accusations aimed at me and my aunt. It made me feel guilty and sad for her. I spent most of my time with her trying to keep her calm. In December, I discovered that going through old family photographs was a distraction that relieved her anxiety.

Mother was terrified by what was happening to her. She presented herself as functional to everyone but me. She feared being thought of as crazy. She talked as little as possible and fought to control herself around other people. When I expressed alarm to other family members about what I was seeing, they felt I was overreacting. They didn't think she was as far out of character as I did, or being anything more than forgetful. My sister felt Mother was very sad and needed to get out more. I felt annoyed, resentful, and alone. I found consolation in talking to friends who had experience caring for elderly parents. I also started praying.

In December, my aunt lost consciousness in church. She was taken to St. Luke's-Roosevelt Hospital Center for observation. They monitored her heart and sent her home.

### 1993: Seeking Help and Advice

In the first six months of 1993, I spent more time visiting Mother and my aunt. I kept my aunt informed about her sister, sought her wisdom, and asked for family history I could talk to Mother about. I discovered my aunt was being treated for high blood pressure. In June, I started looking for help and asking for advice beyond my family and friends. An organization I had taken on as a new client operated a senior citizens' program, and the program's director, with whom I became acquainted, suggested day care for Mother. The director later mailed me an article from the September issue of *McCall's* magazine, "Your Aging Parents: How to Do What's Best and Not Burn Out." *Health* magazine published a special October issue devoted entirely to caring for aging adults. It suggested finding a hospital that offers comprehensive geriatric assessments. I called the New York City Department for the Aging for a referral, and the Mount Sinai Hospital's Department of Geriatrics came highly recommended. In October, I discovered Mother had been taking an anti-depressant since 1987, and I wondered whether it might have something to do with her behavior. My sister mailed me a book by the Public Citizen's Health Research Group, *Worst Pills Best Pills II.* It provided information about the side effects of medications on older adults.

Mother began to weep frequently from the frustration of her condition. She dropped weight because she was losing the ability to feed herself adequately. She took on a dazed look. It became difficult for her to manage her checkbook. In December, Mother fell in the icy snow trying to go to the store by herself.

## 1994: The Problem Gets Defined

Mother strongly resisted, but at her doctor's urging went to Mount Sinai in January 1994. The geriatrician there was very kind. Mother liked her and submitted to examination by a battery of specialists, a psychotherapist, and a psychiatrist. She had a CAT scan and MRIs, and got new glasses. She eventually agreed to stop taking the anti-depressant because the doctors believed that it had lost its effectiveness for her and thought alternatives might produce better results.

In April, my aunt nearly lost consciousness while crossing the street. She was taken to Harlem Hospital Center for observation. They monitored her heart and told me she was dehydrated and had an electrolyte imbalance. Her sister in Washington, DC, died that morning from a massive stroke she had suffered the day before. My aunt asked me to help her with hospital bills, insurance forms, and taxes. I began to routinely escort her to the bank. She was becoming confused and paranoid. It struck me at that time that my mother and aunt were declining, and I began to feel fear and sorrow.

Mother started seeing a psychotherapist in June, which helped her through the process of handing over her independence. Her checks were bouncing because she couldn't fill them out properly, so she gave me her checkbooks. She asked me to hold her cash because she thought some-one was breaking into her apartment and stealing her money. She gradually allowed me to go through her papers to create a file for her private affairs.

In September, it was determined that she had dementia, most likely Alzheimer's disease. I was frightened but relieved to have the problem defined. I read two books on Alzheimer's disease recommended by the therapist and followed his advice to contact the Alzheimer's Association. It became a lifeline for me. I called its hotline many times asking for information and advice, and the people who answered never forgot to ask how I was feeling about what was happening. I attended the Alzheimer's Association's seminars on day care, home care, and long-term care planning. Mother and I attended its seminar on elder law. She was impressed with the guest attorney and allowed me to set up an appointment for a consultation.

Mother was struggling with words. She had 10 percent of the verbal and visual memory of a healthy person her age, and suffered significant loss of cognitive function. I began researching and contacting new resources, and my sister, Mother, and I began to talk about long-term care. Mother denied having Alzheimer's disease. In November she went back to her previous doctor alone. He persuaded her to continue seeing her new doctor. We went to my cousin's house for Thanksgiving dinner. Mother didn't eat because she feared being poisoned. The next day, my cousin took my aunt shopping in New Jersey. She lost consciousness and was hospitalized for observation at Hackensack University Medical Center. They monitored her heart and sent her home. In December, I distributed copies of my research material about Alzheimer's disease, day care, home care, long-term care, and legal considerations to the family.

## 1995: Getting Day Care, Home Care, and Medicaid in Place

By 1995, Mother was pacing at night, constantly wringing her hands, hoarding things, and jumping at noises. She was irrational, incoherent, and having delusions about being watched, and was starting to have difficulty swallowing. She resisted leaving her apartment. I shopped and cooked, straightened and cleaned her apartment, spent some nights with her, secured a durable power of attorney and health care proxy, researched her assets, and looked for private-pay home care. In January, the psychiatrist prescribed a low dose of trazodone for her depression. At first Mother agreed to it, but then resisted; eventually she decided to take it regularly. In February, the therapist confirmed Mother's dementia as Alzheimer's disease, based on the rate of deterioration in her brain. That same month she lost her balance and fell in my apartment. In March, I interviewed home attendants to prepare meals and do light housekeeping. In April, Mother started day care three-and-a-half hours one day a week, which gave me a little time to catch my breath. She slowly started home care a few hours, no more than three days a week.

Mother resisted everything new with tears, even after she had agreed to it. Anything new was a tough challenge for her. I had to be with her, comfort her, and learn a new level of patience. I was dazed by what was happening. I started attending an Alzheimer's Association support group for children of parents with the disease.

In May, I started the application process to the city for Medicaid and home care service. Meanwhile, I hired a home care agency whose attendants were trained to work with Alzheimer's patients. In the last eight months of 1995, Mother adjusted to seven home attendants. They were caring people, but some of them knew less about the disease than I had learned in that short year. The more experienced workers preferred full-time work to a job that lasted four hours a day, four days a week. In June, Mother started taking risperidone for paranoia. The medications worked for her. They reduced some of her symptoms and stopped others, like pacing and wringing her hands. I monitored her pills and watched for side effects.

In August, I created a file of my aunt's personal papers. Her normally neat apartment was in disarray, but she resisted help. In November, Mother's Medicaid was approved, and the City of New York sent a nurse and a social worker to evaluate her need for home care services. By now, Mother didn't know what to do about being hot or cold, nor could she tell you that she was. She needed help to run a bath and dress.

In December, she started attending day care one more day a week at a program for Alzheimer's patients run by the Brookdale Center on Aging of Hunter College. Since Mother didn't identify herself as an Alzheimer's patient, the site coordinator assigned her the position of assistant to the coordinator. After that, she loved going to day care. She was engaged by the culturally sensitive activities, the welcoming hugs from the volunteers, the group games, listening to music, singing gospel songs, and chatting around the lunch table.

This was also a very active year for my business.

## 1996: Mother Enters a Nursing Home

In January 1996, Medicaid sent two doctors to evaluate Mother's need for home care service, and determined that she needed a higher level of care than could be authorized. The doctors suggested that we consider nursing home care. I met with her care team at the Mount Sinai Hospital, talked to our attorney, the Alzheimer's Association, my sister, my aunt, and Mother. I requested a fair hearing to contest the denial of home care services. Meanwhile, her doctor requested services from the Visiting Nurse Service of New York.

Mother was having mini-strokes and other physical emergencies. She burned food, routinely barricaded her door, washed her clothes in bleach, and lost the ability to operate her lock. She could no longer brush her teeth, use the phone, or dress. She was rocking back and forth, having great difficulty communicating, could no longer eat solid foods, and was incontinent. Each new attendant required an orientation period. In April, the Visiting Nurse Service of New York started sending a home health aide to prepare meals, do light housekeeping, and provide personal care six hours a day, six days a week. In the last 11 months of 1996, Mother adjusted to 23 home attendants and home health aides. They needed more training to be able to effectively interact with an Alzheimer's patient. They needed a support group as much as I did. It is very intense and difficult work.

Another MRI showed brain shrinkage and atrophy. The psychiatrist suggested that Mother might be ready for a more structured environment. My sister, Mother, and I talked, and Mother agreed. I started to research, visit, and apply to nursing homes that had special programs for Alzheimer's patients. I didn't think the need for this kind of care would come as soon as it did. It saddened me. I never imagined Mother in a nursing home. Mother was brave about it; home had become a frightening place to be.

In September, my aunt lost consciousness while watching a parade. She was admitted to Harlem Hospital Center for observation. Her best friend, a retired social worker, urged my cousins and me to get her a diagnosis and household help. We held a family meeting with my two cousins, my aunt, and her friend. After the meeting, my aunt allowed me—as Mother previously had—to take her to the Mount Sinai Hospital for a comprehensive geriatric assessment. Later in the year I once again secured a durable power of attorney and health care proxy, and started the application process to the city for Medicaid and home care service.

Mother was accepted by the Hebrew Home for the Aged at Riverdale and put on the waiting list. Meanwhile, the admissions coordinator suggested that she enroll in its day care center. Beginning in October, a van picked her up every day at 8:00 a.m., took her to the Samuels Adult Day Care Center (now known as Elderserve on the Palisades Adult Day Program), and returned her at 4:00 p.m. She had a privately paid home attendant from 4:00 p.m. to 8:00 p.m., and a home health aide from 8:00 p.m. to 8:00 a.m. Under this routine, her condition seemed to improve. Her night home health aide was a very caring and competent person, and Mother thrived at the day care center. Her transfer to the nursing home two days before Thanksgiving, before the fair hearing occurred, went smoothly.

I felt overwhelmed. I had little to no time for business clients, was becoming short-tempered, and had developed a grave medical problem that needed attention. I thought managing my aunt's care would be easier, but it wasn't. I started writing about my feelings and frequently talking to my sister.

### 1997: My Aunt Takes a Turn for the Worse

In 1997, I went about the business of clearing Mother's apartment, observing her care, and managing the transfer of her affairs. In January, my aunt started attending the Samuels Adult Day Care Center two days a week. She was diagnosed with dementia, syncope, and hypertension. She refused further attention to determine if her dementia was Alzheimer's disease. In February, I hired a private-pay home attendant to prepare meals and do light housekeeping eight hours a day, two days a week. In March, Medicaid was approved but home care service was denied. I had laser surgery to remove tumors that feed on estrogen and flourish under stress. I was cared for by two very special friends during the week it took to recover. In April, I requested a fair hearing for home care services. The decision was reevaluated and reversed in May.

My aunt was confused, disoriented, frustrated, and suspicious. She was having difficulty keeping track of her keys and purse. She left the water running in her kitchen. She fell in the hallway of her building. A home care agency under contract to the City of New York started sending a home attendant 18 hours a week; her doctor had requested service eight hours a day, seven days a week. In the last four months of the year, she adjusted to four home attendants.

## 1998: Fighting for Appropriate Home Care

By 1998, Mother was content in her new home, stable, and in good spirits. To reduce the turnover of home attendants, I switched my aunt to a consumer-directed home care agency called Concepts of Independence. It felt like things were settling down, so I started thinking about new career directions. Caregiving had taken so much of my focus that it had forced me to turn down work. I lost most of my clients. At the same time I felt that I couldn't return to a field whose technologies had changed so rapidly in such a short time. I would have to essentially relearn my field and reequip my office.

In June, I changed my aunt's lock because she said someone was breaking into her apartment, stealing, rearranging her belongings, and folding her money. In July, she lost consciousness in her apartment and was revived by her home attendant. Her doctor made a request to the city for home care service 24 hours a day, seven days a week. In August, her service was increased from 18 to 28 hours a week. In September, I changed her lock again. She left the gas on in her kitchen. In October, she lost consciousness in her apartment while she was alone. She was admitted to Mount Sinai for observation. They discharged her nine days later. The next day she lost consciousness on her way to day care and was readmitted to the hospital. She was discharged eight days later. That night she lost consciousness while I was washing her dinner dishes. She was admitted to Mount Sinai a third time.

Her doctor requested 24-hour home care service again. The city increased my aunt's home care from 28 to 55 hours a week. We had another family meeting. My cousins didn't see the need for 24-hour supervision. My aunt wavered on the subject. She agreed that I should start the nursing home application process because waiting for a bed might take a year. Her position all along had been that the more help she received, the more she would need. She cherished her independence. My cousins didn't want to see her lose it. In November, I started spending the night at her place until I could find a private-pay home attendant to work at night. I made sure that someone was with her at all times.

## 1999: A Death in the Family

By December 1998, Mother was fully assisted with all personal care and feeding. She needed a wheelchair for transport during our visits. On New Year's Day, 1999, my aunt lost consciousness in the early morning as she started her day. She was admitted to Harlem Hospital Center for observation. The hospital's request to the city for 24-hour home care service was denied. Near the end of the month, she was transferred from the hospital to the Hebrew Home for the Aged at Riverdale. Mother rallied at the opportunity to visit with her sister.

In June, Mother's doctor asked for a family decision about stomach tube feeding. Dysphagia, combined with the dementia, was sabotaging her ability to swallow enough nourishment to sustain life. When I talked to Mother about the doctor's request, I was grateful that she had the clarity to let me know her choice. She shook her head in disapproval.

Mother lost weight steadily and became confined to a customized wheelchair. By the end of September, she could no longer drink enough liquid to keep herself hydrated, and it became impossible to maintain hydration intravenously because the doctors could not locate her veins. During the last five days of her life she became confined to her bed and was given a special mattress to discourage bedsores. The nurses placed padding around her feet, gave her blankets, propped her up with pillows, and gave her oxygen to keep her comfortable and warm. Her doctor, social worker, and members of the nursing staff regularly came into her room to offer comfort. Her primary nurse's aide had grown to love Mother, so we consoled each other. Several nurse's aides shared their stories with me about the good times they had had with her. They told me how she had recently surprised them with words she had long before lost the ability to say, an outburst of song, and displays of affectionate gratitude for their service. I had noticed that she was strangely joyful in the last few months. She died in early October. I was grateful that I had been in the light of her joy through the struggle of her dying.

My aunt is accustomed to her new home, friendly to her neighbors, and in good humor. My cousins visit her regularly, and her friends visit as well. My life goes on with the peculiar grief known to those who lose a loved one in bits and pieces over a long period of time. I have recognized the trauma of caregiving and am working toward recovery.

Caregiving is enormously stressful. Mine was compounded by excessive paperwork, widespread misinformation about Alzheimer's disease among the general public, and huge city bureaucracies long on caring individuals and short on accurate communications. Most distressing was hearing health care workers and city employees refer to the disease as just memory loss that requires more patience. It is so much more than that.

I am thankful to the individuals, professionals, and organizations that taught me how to care for an Alzheimer's patient. Caregivers need support to survive. We need support to keep caring. I am very grateful to the many people too numerous to mention here who were genuinely helpful to me over this decade. You have widened my heart and given me strength.

My story is one of many. I was drawn into this life experience kicking and screaming inside, but with a commitment to honor my family heritage and my own strong personal belief that family members should care for one another. It brought me closer to my mother, aunt, family, and friends. I learned a lot about my family and myself. I grew closer to my God. People from my community kept telling me I would be blessed for what I was doing. I feel like I was blessed by the doing.

I have been privileged to share my story with you in this book. My hope is that it helps to motivate change, that it may inspire individuals to support legislation, organizations, policies, practices, and efforts to improve services to elders and caregivers.

# 3

# A Crisis of Caregiving, a Crisis of Faith

*Rabbi Gerald I. Wolpe*


## I. 2000: The First 14 Years

On April 10, 1986, at 11:05 in the evening, my wife collapsed in our home from the rupture of two brain aneurysms. That began a phantasmagoria of events that has since determined the structure of our lives. In a traumatic second she went from being an articulate public speaker, college administrator, teacher, and extraordinary wife and mother to a severely damaged woman. In the past 14 years she has defied almost every statistic. Few people survive the level of cerebral damage she sustained. If, by some miracle, they do survive, the extent of brain damage that usually accompanies the rupture of a brain aneurysm, let alone two bleeding centers, results in severe cognitive disruption.

The attending physicians predicted that Elaine's death was certain and imminent. But after weeks in a coma she awoke, only to face overwhelming challenges. She was diagnosed with severe expressive Broca's aphasia. She had the typical symptoms of this form of aphasia, which for years impaired her ability to speak except for occasional utterances of a nonsense syllable. Though she was cognitively sound, able to understand spoken language, and physically whole, her inability to transmit her thoughts into words, spoken or written, frustrated her constantly. A remarkable and determined woman, she has battled valiantly to adjust to this brutal, daily challenge.

While this catastrophe struck her directly, it happened to our family as well. We are the parents of four sons, each of whom has made a major mark in his field. We were living a wonderful life of public service and commitment to our own careers. Everything seemed to be unfolding according to a well-designed plan when the façade collapsed. We were a public family, living in the spotlight of congregational and community activity, and our agony was not to be a private affair.

## Managing the Immediate Crisis

In the beginning, loyal friends and concerned supporters rallied to my side, flooding the hospital. Eventually, hospital staff members asked me to restrict the number of visitors as there was not enough room for all of them. Day and night, people would visit and ask, "What can we do for you, Rabbi?"

Through it all I was truly indefatigable. My adrenaline flowed as I conferred with physicians, comforted family members, and made important medical decisions on Elaine's behalf. In no way do I wish to make light of the situation, because it was horrible, but it was an incredible drama. I listened to the flood of medical advice from physicians in my congregation. We had over 2,000 members in our synagogue and a sizable number of them were doctors. They provided invaluable help in managing Elaine's clinical condition and suggesting referrals to the best available specialists. That outpouring of support remains one bright note in a period of intense stress and despair.

Then I began to hear disturbing advice. Over and over my congregants would tell me, "Rabbi, be strong. God will be good." I said to myself, "If God were so good, why did this happen in the first place? What did Elaine do to deserve this?" I discovered that I was relying on the great philosopher Woody Allen, who once said that God is an underachiever. "Rabbi, you give us strength," they would say. All the while I was screaming inside for someone to help me. So it was not only a crisis of practical response, it was a crisis of faith at a time when everyone expected me to be the symbol of unwavering faith. I was the rabbi and I was supposed to set the example for the best possible way to handle this trial.

## A Caregiver without Training

I am still amazed that I was able to watch myself, almost from a detached perspective, as I tried to make sense of the unfolding horror. It should have come as no surprise, because I supposedly had all the proper credentials to be a caregiver. As a rabbi I have counseled many people. I have been on the faculty of three medical schools and have a specialty in medical sociology and bioethics. I had spent years on ethics review boards that dealt with research and clinical protocols. I had lectured extensively on the relationship of the health care community to patients and family members. I assumed, therefore, that I was somewhat sophisticated and knowledgeable about the health care delivery system. Who else would be so well prepared to be a caregiver? Still, it was a disaster.

I found myself bewildered and under total emotional siege. Even though I had, in my classroom, inveighed against the passivity of patients and caregivers, I found myself accepting, all too readily, the comfort of leaving decisions to the doctors. It was so much easier to be lulled by the authority of the health care professional. I had to battle constantly to maintain my sense of perspective and a modicum of control. This became more of an issue as my wife's acute condition settled into a chronic state over months and years. An emotional fatigue gripped me and required that I call for more outside help and advice. At the same time, though, I realized that the basic decisions were mine. As much as I wanted relief from the constant onslaught of responsibilities, it was my mandate to be in charge.

In retrospect, I realize that I had been thrust into the role of caregiver without any preparation. None of the health professionals caring for my wife, nor any of the doctors in my congregation, ever told me how to manage the transition from emergency to long-term illness, from being a husband to also being a caregiver. Acute illness is clearly defined by time and clinical activity. Chronic illness entails a daily regimen that has no time parameters. This transition is still happening 14 years later.

When the immediate crisis subsided, people who we considered among our closest friends disappeared. They were unwilling to adjust to the sudden change in our lives. That phenomenon seems to be common for people who experience dramatic shifts: those who become widowed; couples who divorce or separate; and those who become chronically ill or disabled. When a serious injury or illness renders an individual unrecognizable, many friends are unwilling to make the emotional adjustment necessary to continue the relationship. These losses can lead to feelings of disillusionment, betrayal, and loneliness. We were no exception.

With all of my experience and supposed sophistication, I realized I had to learn a new vocabulary. Before my wife's collapse I had never heard of aphasia. As I was introduced to clinical therapies for my wife's condition, which were almost primitive in 1986, I learned the technique of tonal intonation. A therapist had discovered that the brain processes speech and music in different areas. While aphasics' abilities to put their thoughts into words are damaged, the therapist found that they might eventually be able to regain speech ability by reciting words as *recitative*. Since the portion of Elaine's brain that processes music was not damaged, I used the technique to reintroduce language to her. The technique helped her think about words in song and, eventually, express herself, albeit in a limited fashion. I became an expert in responding to aphasia, not by study alone but by the trial of a beloved.

How devastating it was in those early years to talk and listen to someone who had been so articulate yet whose speech was now limited to an unintelligible syllable. In the first two years after she became ill, she was able to articulate only one word I could understand: "prison." She was in a prison of verbal isolation. In many ways I was also in prison, a prison of existential horror—the prison of caregiving. We had been companions in so many ways. We had a loving marriage of giving and sharing. We had a relationship of care, admiration, and concern. We depended on each other's talents for mutual support and growth. Now I was required to be the decision maker. At a time when I needed her strength and sagacity as never before, she was in the midst of her own battle against an indescribable isolation that required all of her energy and resiliency.

There were other issues, which I can talk about only now, more than 14 years after that chilling moment. I wasn't prepared for the role reversal, a man caregiving for a woman. On one particularly upsetting occasion I found myself screaming at my wife's gynecologist on the phone, "What do I do?" I had been married to her for over 30 years and I had no idea how her body functioned. A woman's gynecological needs, daily and monthly, are handled by her in discreet privacy and not before her husband. Now it was my responsibility.

## Seeking Support

In the midst of all of these imponderables, one of my sons said to me, "Dad, you have it so much easier than we do." I was taken aback. "What are you talking about?" I asked. "You only have to worry about Mother," he said. "We're worried about both of you." My sons insisted that I see a therapist. I did and realized that, after about a half-hour, he was telling me his problems. After all, I was a rabbi and it was my function to listen to problems. I told him, "I don't have to pay you $125 an hour to hear your problems. I listen to problems all day long." That was my first cautious step into therapy. The second, a more challenging one as it had a certain philosophical impact, occurred when a psychiatrist said to me, "Rabbi, let me ask you a question. If someone came to you with this problem, what would you say?" That was a shattering cold moment. I knew that he was saying to me, "You know the answer as well as I do." I did not realize at the time that what I really needed was just to let loose. I just needed to be able to cry, to be able to scream.

In 1991 I discovered a helpful source of support, the Well Spouse Foundation. Its motto explains its mission: "When one person is ill, two need help." That group was vital, not only for mutual support with fellow caregivers but also for helping me develop a vocabulary to understand what I was experiencing. Before I encountered Well Spouse, I had never heard of the term "caregiver." I realized that the group had already begun to articulate the existential issues with which I was grappling but had not yet put into words. I learned that I was part of a defined category of people, while at the same time I was struggling as an individual to make some sense and purpose out of a dramatic life change. Well Spouse helped me identify that I was on a separate, but parallel, path from Elaine, a path with its own distinct challenges. Caregivers are a group that has always existed but had just begun the process of self-identification and -definition.

## Caregiving Takes Its Toll

Recently I realized that, for years, I had turned emotionally inward in an attempt to maintain control. I banked many of my emotions in the name of efficiency. I internalized my own sorrow, anger, frustration, and fear for the sake of my wife, who was battling her own inner struggles. It took its toll. Six years ago I had a heart attack.

The health conditions of caregivers are rarely discussed. We become ill as a result of the stress we experience. Primary caregivers provide an average of more than 20 hours of care per week, and many provide 40 hours or more. Almost a quarter have been providing care for five to nine years, and another quarter for ten years or more. This amounts to an almost constant state of caregiving (Donelan et al. 2002). Their clinical status is even starker: caregivers are more likely to experience health problems due to caregiving, and some face the risk of serious illness, including cardiac problems (Rabin 1999; Glassman and Shapiro 1998; Kiecolt-Glaser et al. 1996; Shaw et al. 1997). I am part of that statistic. Most disturbing of all, older caregivers who experience emotional or mental strain are at greater risk of dying (Schulz and Beach 1999).

As I lay in the intensive care unit and listened to the pronouncements of the cardiac surgeon, I was beset with a familiar bifurcation of emotions. Of course, I was worried about myself. This was an attack on my mortality. I was to undergo emergency bypass surgery. My life was in danger and

I was frightened. At the same time, Elaine was on my mind. Who would take care of her? Our sons and their wives are extraordinarily attentive, but they have their own lives. No one would take care of her as I had throughout these years. At that moment of ultimate personal challenge, I did not even have the time to luxuriate in my own health crisis. Elaine sat by my bed and held my hand. I could see the fear in her eyes; she was worried about me. She later told me that she could see the fear in my eyes. I was worried about the two of us.

## A Universal Problem

As former First Lady Rosalynn Carter said, there are only four kinds of people in the world: those who have been caregivers, those who are currently caregivers, those who will be caregivers, and those who will need caregivers. This makes caregiving a universal problem.

If this is true, then how can we better prepare caregivers to enter this role? I have heard the suggestion that caregivers should make their needs better known. Most caregivers struggle with this advice because it takes time for them to recognize that they *are* caregivers. In addition, caregiving consumes so much of the day that caregivers rarely have the time to seek help from outside sources.

If caregivers did seek assistance, where would they begin? With health care professionals? God help them if they do, because health care professionals work in institutional settings and generally provide little assistance to help people make the transition to the role of caregiver. For most of the health care community, the emphasis is on the patient, and the family caregiver is visible only as a surrogate for the ill family member. Caregivers' needs are rarely on health care professionals' agendas, but the fact is that they need support as much as do patients.

Should they seek help from social service organizations? The social service community is just becoming aware of caregivers' circumstances, and has yet to respond with adequate support services. Any programs these organizations create must have the flexibility to meet the varied needs of caregivers as patients move through different stages of illness. More importantly, services must be developed to support caregivers through the long periods when their ill or disabled loved ones remain in a steady, chronic state.

How about the clergy? There are no rituals for caregiving. There are traditional and modern rituals and liturgies for dying, but not for caregiving. And what are you going to pray for? Traditional pastoral care has tended to view the caregiver only in relationship to the ill family member. Religious leaders and secular counselors possess little understanding of caregivers' needs.

In 1998 I completed the text for a book called *Mrs. Job: Caregiver in the Shadows.* Has anyone ever thought about Mrs. Job? The book of Job tells the story of a good man who suffers the onslaught of disease and the loss of everything he values, including his children. Mrs. Job watches her husband suffer and lives through these losses, but no one comes to comfort her. Only one statement is attributed to her in the book. She says to her husband, "Curse God and die!" Throughout the years, commentators have condemned her statement as the ultimate blasphemy. But I understand what she's saying: "Let me out of here. I want an end to it." It is the cry of desperation.

The emotional drain on caregivers can indeed be intense. There is an unrelenting progression of exhaustion, anger, isolation, and resentment, mixed with guilt over having these feelings about someone you love but whose condition has nevertheless bound you in a daily emotional prison. Day after day, caregiving also involves financial management. Chronic illness creates horrendous financial hemorrhaging; philosophy, theology, and even skill in complex home care fade in significance before the dismaying onslaught of financial strain. Perhaps the most frightening part of all is watching one's life's accumulated treasures disappear.

## Small Victories

The years since Elaine became ill have featured daily challenges with the constant strain of her needs and the mourning of the end of previous expectations. But Elaine has made some remarkable progress. Intensive therapy helped her regain some language skills. She can speak in short phrases, achieved by a tremendous amount of effort. Her writing hand is immobile, but she can write with her other hand, however illegibly. She can read a newspaper or a detective novel, although her concentration is limited. She has a specially outfitted automobile, which allows her precious individual mobility. As with all aphasics, life is tremendously frustrating. While cognitively acute, she still struggles with self-expression.

Amid the trials of the last 14 years, there have also been the marriage of our sons, the birth of grandchildren, and public recognition for professional achievement. Elaine, with her verve and talent, founded a unique aphasia center at a rehabilitation hospital in Philadelphia, which has become a prototype for other needed centers. My own work with health care and bioethics has been a salve for the emotional battering that has characterized these years. Our greatest collective success has been in the ability to help identify caregivers as worthy of attention of the health care, religious, political, and media communities. It is no longer the lonely battle it once was to expand awareness and to effect response. This book is an example of that victory.

On my desk I have a picture of my wife holding her first grandchild for the first time. Ariel is looking at her grandmother, who is as much a miracle as is she. I keep it before me as a reminder that success is multileveled. Some questions were answered; some are still shrouded in silence and have yet to be voiced. The fact that there are still questions to be asked and answered is the greatest hope of all.

## II. Three Years Later: Where Has All the Resiliency Gone?

*It is now 17 years since I became a caregiver. These are some of my reflections on the experiences of the three years since the original essay was published.*

I have not had a casual conversation with my wife in 17 years. Aphasia has its own rules for the caregiver. I must not move my eyes, I must not interrupt or try to help during hesitancies, I must not ask complex questions, I must not show impatience, I must not overlook the noise level in the room, I must not speak in a normal cadence. "I must not" has been the constant theme. Every day, I must not, I must not . . .

Each disease has its own rules, but all caregivers have a common challenge. Being identified only with the patient and her needs results in a constant crisis of self-identity. How often I hear, "You must take care of yourself; Elaine needs you." That, of course, is true. My strength is vital to her well-being. Still, I secretly yearn for an expression of concern for me, just for me.

The number of people who remember Elaine before her brain injury is dwindling. The powerful desire to describe her previous vivacity and brilliance is directed at an expanding audience. Yet there is an inspiring magnificence in her struggle and a continuing charm that has captured me for over 50 years.

Our granddaughters sit enthralled, watching a videotape of Elaine at their parents' wedding. How articulate she was as she expressed her blessings for her children! The girls move closer to their Bubbe, hug her, smile, and talk about what they have seen. Not having known the Elaine that was, they love the Bubbe that is.

My desire, my *need*, to maintain some independence is a constant. Yet attending to each career demand requires planning. Can I accept a prestigious out-of-town lecture invitation and leave my wife alone? Are my children available for emergency calls? Will her erratic requests for help disturb my preparations? Will she remember to wear her alarm bracelet? Will the home helper arrive on time? Will I be able to concentrate on my conference, if I do go, as I continually glance at the omnipresent cell phone? My doctor suggests that I reconsider my crowded calendar. The demands are beginning to take their toll. He is correct, but I recognize that each step means retreat, retrenching, and also surrender.

The aphorism rises from the page. "Life is what happens to you when you are making other plans."

Yiddish is the only language, to my knowledge, that has a separate verb for each kind of pain. Yet there is no verb for the deep fatigue and pain that is integral to caregiving. It is not just the hours or the tasks. It comes from a brutal inner struggle. What resentments am I allowed without being uncaring? What resistance am I allowed to her requests without being cruel? What can I demand for myself without being egocentric? What can I dream about without being unrealistic? At first, the task was defining questions. After seventeen years it is the struggle to answer them.

The medical students are polite; their notebooks are open and their pens poised. Caregiving has become an accepted subject. My lecture combines fact and anecdote. Inevitably, the students' questions become autobiographical, informed by caregiving challenges within their own families. Their stories are familiar and they feel free to criticize the profession they are about to enter. The medical response or lack of response in their family's experience shapes their perspective. They have made a major leap into detached concern. No matter the specialty they pursue, I hope they will recognize the family as part of the healing process. Today, they have given caregiving de facto recognition.

Yogi Berra said it well: "It's déjà vu all over again." Seventeen years almost to the day of Elaine's first surgery, the neurosurgeon must again enter the mysterious labyrinth of her brain. Repair work is necessary. It is the same waiting, the same dread, the same false bravery with family. Yet I can feel the difference. I am older and my staying power has ebbed. I know the scenario well and this time there is no comfort from naiveté.

Why have both challenges appeared just before Passover? Is this crisis designed to have the entire family sit together, not just for the Seder, but also for the hours of hospital waiting?

Elaine is wheeled back to her room. Once again, she has survived. The side of her head has been shaved. Much of her beautiful hair, of which she is so proud, has been removed. I bend to kiss her and tell her about the loss. She smiles and says, "Mohawk." The family's nervous smiles become an outburst of spontaneous laughter. She is still the remarkable survivor. But she is older and the strain is obvious. I too am older, and less resilient.

The routine begins again—the same but different, as it bears the emotional weight of seventeen years. Laughter and tears, gratitude and concern, resolve and unease, therapists and calendar time, health insurance and financial planning, constant requests and needs, negotiating the maze of the medical system, endless scheduling of medical tests and supervision, resetting a calendar to fit in my own professional and personal schedule, the search for the respite of my own emotional territory, my prayers of gratitude and my prayers for strength. The acute stage, once again, was easy. Now, it is back to caregiving. It's déjà vu all over again.

The words of the poet Yeats challenge me constantly: "Too long a sacrifice can make a stone of the heart." It is a daily struggle to make certain that the heart remains supple and responsive. In a dramatic moment, aneurysms burst and my wife suddenly became a stranger. The ensuing seventeen years have seen the daily reintroduction to a loved one who is the same person but so different. In many ways, I have become a stranger as well. Medicine can define her condition; other disciplines struggle to identify and define me, the caregiver. I am grateful that I am finally accepted as a partner in the drama. But the recognition of whom I have become as a caregiver is a lonely existential challenge, an ancient struggle for self-identity—a constant rejection, by love and commitment, of the petrifaction of my heart.

## References

Donelan K, CA Hill, C Hoffman, K Scoles, PH Feldman, C Levine, and D Gould. 2002. Challenged to care: Informal caregivers in a changing health system. *Health Affairs (Millwood)* 21(4): 222-31.

Glassman AH and PA Shapiro. 1998. Depression and the course of coronary artery disease. *American Journal of Psychiatry* 155(1): 4-11.

Kiecolt-Glaser JK, R Glaser, S Gravenstein, WB Malarkey, and J Sheridan. 1996. Chronic stress alters the immune response to influenza virus vaccine in older adults. *Proceedings from the National Academy of Sciences USA* 93(7): 3043-7.

Rabin BS. 1999. *Stress, immune function, and health: The connection.* New York: Wiley-Liss and Sons.

Schulz R and SR Beach. 1999. Caregiving as a risk factor for mortality: The Caregiver Health Effects Study. *Journal of the American Medical Association* 282(23): 2215-19.

Shaw WS, TL Patterson, SJ Semple, S Ho, MR Irwin, RL Hauger, and I Grant. 1997. Longitudinal analysis of multiple indicators of health decline among spousal caregivers. *Annals of Behavioral Medicine* 19(2): 101-9.

# 4     Learning to Be a Caregiver, Trying to Be a Brother

*Timothy J. Sweeney*

      My brother Mark disclosed his HIV-positive status to me at Sam's Falafel House in Greenwich Village in 1986. We had just sat down for lunch when he blurted out the news and started to weep quietly. We were gay men living in New York City in the 1980s, so the threat of the AIDS virus was quite real, but now it was hitting our family. After lunch we both went back to work, but later that night I went to visit Mark and ended up holding him in bed all night. I don't know which one of us needed reassurance more. I wanted to save my brother more than anything in the world.

      Seven years later he died alone in his bed at New York Hospital. He had received excellent care, but the disease had ravaged his body, leaving him blind and weighing barely 90 pounds. On the night of his death, I was on a train coming back from Washington, DC, where I was working on the Clinton health care reform plan. I didn't realize it at the time, but Mark chose to die that day, knowing I wouldn't be there. He had always said that our separation was the most difficult thing for him to consider. Somehow leaving this world in my absence must have made that unbearable good-bye easier to face.

      My brother and I were very close. We grew up in Billings, Montana, sharing a bedroom for 16 years, two of seven siblings paired off in a large Irish Catholic family. We had shared the trials and joys of coming out, and we purposely lived close to each other. We were each other's favorite audience, and time spent together was as comfortable as an old pair of jeans. My brother worked in theater and film and, if he put in enough hours in a given quarter, had health insurance. When he died he was working on the children's television program *Ghostbusters*. Earlier that year I had left my job as executive director of Gay Men's Health Crisis (GMHC), the nation's oldest and largest AIDS service, education, and advocacy organization, to care for him. I was a nationally known and respected advocate and helped shape many local, state, and national AIDS policies and programs. The true test of my skills, however, was in caregiving for my brother. In fact, it became a second job.

Being the primary caregiver for my brother, I consciously and unconsciously assumed many roles. At various points I felt like a nurse and doctor, counselor and friend, care team manager, and insurance specialist and banker. I was the executor of his estate and had medical and financial powers of attorney. In the end, I found out that the most important thing I could be was just his brother.

## Nurse and Doctor

Before Mark got sick I hadn't had much direct personal contact with the health care system. I had helped care for other gay male friends who had AIDS, but never to this extent. I really had no idea of the scope of what I would have to do. After one of his earlier hospitalizations, my brother came home with a Hickman catheter implanted in his chest, which was used to administer the medications he needed throughout the day. To begin with, the process involves using needles, which I hate. But then bubbles would get in the line and the whole electronic system would start to beep loudly. Sometimes just flicking the line with my finger would get the bubbles to move on, but other times nothing seemed to work. Our back-up plan, if the eight-hour-a-day home care attendant was not present, was to call a toll-free number and get coached over the phone. Of course, when that didn't work the tension and frustration would boil over. My brother wanted to handle most of his care himself, but as he lost his eyesight, he couldn't see the tubes, needles, or bubbles. But he could hear the beeping, and he would just rage at why we were expected to handle this procedure at home. I would try to calm him down, but inside I would be screaming, "Why am I doing this? I'm not a nurse or a doctor!" On the other hand, neither of us wanted him to be back in the hospital.

Even when he was in the hospital, there were times when I felt totally unprepared. When Mark's catheter got infected, the doctor recommended that it be removed and a second one implanted. He assured us it would be a simple procedure, and when Mark asked if I could stay with him through it, the doctor said fine. There I stood next to Mark, holding him while this amazing surgeon took out a blade and removed the catheter. I was stunned and nauseated as I watched this piece of equipment emerge from my brother's chest. I almost vomited. Meanwhile, Mark was looking to me for support and reassurance. Finally the procedure ended and the doctor proclaimed it a success, which I tried to convey to my brother to comfort him. When the doctor left us alone in the room I gathered my thoughts and realized I wanted to rail at him: "Why didn't you tell me what surgery would be like?" For the doctor it was routine, but for me it was my brother's chest.

## Counselor and Friend

Later in my brother's illness he started to have hallucinations, so my partner, Jay, and I brought him to stay at our apartment. Mark would wake up in the middle of the night and, despite his weakened state, pace back and forth in the living room. He wrote poems and produced drawings prolifically. The poems and the drawings were often about AIDS, the doctors, the drugs he took for his illness, and his life. Some nights he would produce as many as thirty drawings and dozens of poems. It didn't occur to me that this was abnormal or might require intervention. I thought he was dying. He had told me he wanted to die at home, so I thought I was doing the right thing by supporting his drawing and writing. He would, however, get very manic and scared, which made me nervous. Our apartment is on the seventeenth floor of a high-rise building and I was worried he would jump off the balcony. Jay and I would invite Mark to sleep in our bed between us, which seemed to bring him some relief from his fears and demons.

One night he woke up and told me he had had a beautiful dream that butterflies had come to take him away. I thought he was dying right then and there, but he only fell asleep. When he woke up later he described in intricate, exacting detail a memory from childhood that I had completely forgotten. It was of a florist's window in our town that we would stare at for hours, mesmerized by the tropical flowers and lush greenery that seemed so exotic to us in arid, sparsely vegetated southeastern Montana.

There were times during this period when I thought my brother was mystical and was maybe showing me things that I was privileged to see. Needless to say, my partner didn't sleep very well those nights, though he was, as usual, very patient and even wrote a song for my brother about the butterfly dream. After one particularly acute episode of hallucinations, I woke up exhausted, but nonetheless started the Sunday morning by offering to make French toast (my brother's favorite breakfast). My brother looked right at me and said, "I think I need some help. You can't handle this manic behavior." I was stunned. It hadn't occurred to me that I should call the doctor.

When we did call the doctor, he immediately saw my brother and gave him medication for the hallucinations. But the treatment didn't work well for Mark, and his hallucinations continued. So I felt I had no choice: I had Mark admitted to the Payne-Whitney Psychiatric Clinic. That was one of the hardest days of my life because my brother felt I had abandoned and betrayed him by leaving him in a hospital with locked doors. He was petrified of the spinal tap they would have to perform as part of the testing procedures, and he deeply resented the medical residents who came by to review his case. On the second day when I visited him, he threw a pile of books at me and told me to quit being so damned optimistic and to stop making plans for the future. Later when my brother would call me from the floor pay phone, I would feel guilty because I had brought him to a place he despised and which he couldn't get out of, but most of all because I couldn't do anything to help him.

On the other hand, Mark found one of his greatest doctors in that hospital. This psychiatrist became a key support not only for Mark but also for my sister and me, because he taught us a system for checking in with each other—in a formal, conscious, respectful session where we talked about what was on each other's minds and really listened to one another. It soon became clear that we all had unmet needs and were confused about our roles. My brother liked these check-in sessions because it helped alleviate the constant sense of guilt he felt about being a burden on us. They provided him with a way to help us by strategizing how we could all take care of ourselves.

## Care Team Manager

One of the most challenging aspects of being the primary caregiver for my brother was managing the team of people who wanted to help take care of him. This team included my sister, Lib, who moved from Seattle to New York to be with my brother and to support me. She became, in essence, my co-partner in my brother's care for the last two years of his life. It took me months to realize that my sister came to New York to help *me*. She has amazing emotional strength and quite a bit more experience with the health care system. It was hard at first to let my sister take on some of the primary caregiving duties because I felt I was letting my brother down, but he was in fact very glad Lib was there for him and me. More than anyone else, Lib taught me to understand and respect my and Mark's limits when it came to caregiving. She taught me how and when to give up control and let events take their course. I wish all caregivers could have someone like Lib to help them through—someone who can assist them when they don't know they need assistance, and someone to tell them they can't do everything and determine every outcome.

A catastrophic illness brings up many questions about the relationships one has in life. Many of my brother's greatest needs centered on settling his feelings about his past relationships and friendships. In addition to Lib and me, Mark had a large group of friends and acquaintances who wanted to help him. I tried to encourage Mark to determine who he wanted to be part of his caregiving team, because I knew how important it was for him to maintain as much control over his life as possible. Yet I found his behavior very perplexing. At times my brother seemed mercurial, mean, or inscrutable toward these people. He sometimes refused their offers to help. He rebuffed attempts at reconciliation. But then there were other times when he was very open to offers of support, love, and friendship. All I could do was accept that he had his own journey to complete and sit back and watch.

Some friends were great for a while, but as my brother became sicker, they just disappeared. AIDS had taken such a toll on my brother's circle that it didn't surprise me that some people just gave up or were in denial. On the other hand, some people really came through with just the right touch—with visits and conversations, calls, cookies, or flowers. Some work colleagues continued giving Mark professional updates, knowing how much my brother valued his career. Some old friends and lovers helped Mark achieve major breakthroughs and avert crises at times when he simply couldn't accept help from me.

Once my brother just lost control emotionally and went wandering along 14th Street at four o'clock in the morning to find an old acquaintance. I still shudder to think what could have happened to him at that hour with his terrible eyesight. But his friend took him in, calmed him down, gave him a bed to sleep in, and brought him home the next day. Over brunch one day another couple helped Mark face the fact that he had to quit working and really take care of himself. It was a very difficult, tearful conversation that morning, one which I had been trying to have with him for more than a year. Days like that helped me accept the fact that he couldn't hear everything from me, that difficult conversations would sometimes just have to wait until he was ready, and that when we finally had them, he might need a listening ear more than anything else.

## Family Ties

My relationship with my blood family was even more complicated. I kept my brother's HIV diagnosis a secret for many years until he decided to tell my parents, which for me, as an AIDS advocate, was very difficult. Later in his illness he went to Montana and told them, and it was a great relief to him that they responded with love and concern. However, like many gay men, we had had limited communication with our family over the years. My parents had struggled with our homosexuality and now they had to deal with their son's HIV disease. I tried to be respectful of our blood family's needs and concerns, but when we disagreed about what was best for Mark I felt the need to protect him.

Fortunately, our family really came through for him. I was conscious of how every member of our family, all four other siblings and some of my in-laws, tried to follow my sister's example and support Mark as best they could. This support came in the form of their numerous visits to New York City. In my large family it is always difficult to get time alone with each other, but that is so important when issues of life and death present themselves. I was also keenly aware that my dad, being a lawyer, probably wanted to give me advice about how best to advocate for my brother around his insurance and financial issues.

I knew the spiritual aspects of my parents' life made it very important for them to have my brother make some reconciliation with the Catholic Church. Mark was a lapsed Catholic but was very spiritual in his own private way. We had had numerous conversations about his views on religion and he told me he did not want any religious ceremonies before or after his death. At the end of his life when my parents visited for the last time, however, my mother expressed her strong desire for my brother to have a sacrament known as the Last Rites. I worried that my parents were manipulating him and I tried to intervene. It was so difficult to see my mom struggle over the appropriate role for her in saving her son's soul. She and my father were keenly aware of the Catholic Church's shortcomings on issues of sexuality and AIDS. They had even become active back in Montana in their faith community to raise consciousness about AIDS and provide care for those with HIV.

It therefore came as quite a surprise when I learned that my brother had decided to accept Last Rites. It taught me another lesson about the unpredictability of being a caregiver: you may think that you know your loved one's wishes, but they can completely change without any prior warning. Working with the hospital's chaplain, my parents made the extra effort to find a gay-friendly priest who blessed my brother and asked his forgiveness of the church for its homophobia and AIDS phobia. I admire my parents and my brother for working to find common spiritual ground. I also felt so lucky to have found this chaplain, who became a critical part of the care team. She helped my sister and me determine the best times to have family members visit Mark. She helped us understand some of the limits of my brother's treatment options. She gave my parents practical advice about where to get a cup of coffee and lunch and the closest Catholic church for a prayer and rosary. She helped humanize New York for a couple from Billings that was not familiar with the city.

## Insurance Specialist and Banker

Helping manage my brother's health insurance claims presented its own set of difficulties and placed me in yet another role as caregiver: insurance specialist and banker. By the time I got involved, the flood of paperwork had already become overwhelming. I felt like I was intruding and controlling my brother's life when I started to handle his finances. He prided himself on his independence, and there I found myself poring over his checkbook, filling out reimbursement claims, making mistakes, and generally doing a terrible job of it all. We had to work with his union local, which was another bureaucracy to master. Finally, my brother had to spend down all his assets to qualify for Medicaid. Thankfully he became a client of the city-financed Division of AIDS Services (DAS) program, which paid his rent. The process to keep him certified and make sure the landlord received the rent check every month was horrendous, however. Many of the DAS workers were untrained and overworked. My brother and I spent hours on the phone and going to the DAS office to complete paperwork or ensure payments had been processed. Mark received numerous eviction notices, but fortunately the Legal Services department of Gay Men's Health Crisis prevented them from taking effect.

I wanted my brother to have a good quality of life, so when it was necessary I spent money out of my own pocket. Whether it was for cab rides up the East River Drive to the hospital or special take-out food that might put some weight on him, I didn't care how much it would cost. We even took a very special trip to see my brother in Thailand. Soon I realized I was spending down my savings, but I was lucky because my partner, Jay, provided financial backup. This helped me make the crucial decision to leave my job at GMHC and concentrate on my brother. I started a consulting business out of my home, and the flexibility it provided proved priceless in the last year of my brother's life. I was no longer the CEO of a high-profile, $23 million dollar agency with 220 staff, 2,000 volunteers, and 5,000 clients. Better yet, I could work on health care policy, which helped me focus my anger and activism. Most importantly, I had the time to just be with my brother, to quietly read to him, or give him a foot massage or a shave. I think I finally listened to all the advice people had been giving me: I allowed myself to slow down and relax. Many of my family members visited Mark and we had several meaningful family gatherings during that time. I even got time off to go with my partner for a week-long Christmas vacation while Mark was with my family in Montana.

## Flying toward the Sun

The last day I saw my brother he was on morphine. He was lucid, tired, and seemed peaceful except for the pain. My sister and I had been visiting him in the hospital every day, sometimes twice a day. I think I was in denial at that point, just refusing to believe my brother could die. That day he and I reminisced about a game of chase our family played a couple of Christmases before on the frozen lake by our cabin. It was the last Christmas our whole family was together, and we laughed like kids as we slid all over the ice trying to catch each other. When I left that day he was getting drowsy so I bent down to kiss him and he kissed me back and whispered in my ear as he jabbed me with his finger, "You're it." I said, "Oh god, you got me." He said, "Now go to Washington and get that national health plan passed. We all need it." I told him I would be back tomorrow on the late afternoon train and would come up to see him. He just nodded and told me he loved me. That was the last conversation we ever had.

My brother was cremated and we spread his ashes up at the lake by our family's cabin in Montana and by the Delacorte Theater in Central Park, following his wishes. The October day we chose to spread his ashes in Montana turned out to be gloriously beautiful. We hiked to the cabin and canoed to the center of the lake where we formed an improvised grieving circle. We managed to quiet ourselves down so we could each contemplate for a while, and then we tossed Mark's ashes into the crystal clear water.

My parents organized a funeral mass in Billings that reflected the healing spirit that they had achieved with my brother. They demanded, and won, the right to have a special priest who was supportive of their AIDS work concelebrate the mass. My older brother gave a eulogy that clearly expressed the pride our family felt in my gay brother. The obituary in the local paper mentioned AIDS as the cause of death, referred to my brother as an openly gay man, and included a picture of Mark. The obituary sparked an outpouring of support from the community, and my parents received hundreds of supportive letters and cards. They still are active in caring for people with HIV disease and educating people about AIDS stigma and homophobia.

My family's leadership around the funeral was a great source of healing for me, because I was simply too exhausted at that point. My brother and his wife came to New York City and helped me empty Mark's apartment and organize his final bills. Their practical help kept me from getting physically sick and gave me the boost I needed to handle all the estate matters.

Mark's chosen family in New York gave a memorial service for him in the West Village. His friends created shrines with photos of his works of art and poems. We had lots of open storytelling, food, and drink. It was an amazing mix of people from his scattered life, and it finally helped me feel like this journey he and I took together was over for a while. We drank a final toast and danced to Petula Clark singing "Downtown." My parents later published a book of my brother's poetry and made a panel for the AIDS quilt following the design of one of his collages he made while in the hospital. The collage was a blackbird trying to get free and fly toward the sun.

# 5 Pushing the Boundaries in Assisted Living: Failures in Caring

*Robert L. Kane and Joan C. West*

Not all caregiving occurs at home. Nor does family caregiving stop when a person is institutionalized. This chapter describes the dilemmas and frustrations facing us, two adult children attempting to look after our mother when she suffered cognitive impairment following a stroke. One of us, Robert, is a nationally known geriatrician who has researched and written extensively on long-term care; the other, Joan, is a master's-prepared elementary school teacher. We were experienced and savvy, we'd thought, and had the advantage of working as a team. If we, with our resources and knowledge, found dealing with the long-term care system difficult, what chance has the ordinary family caregiver?

## The First Transition

Our mother had always taken great pride in her independence. Her greatest fear was that of becoming disabled. On numerous occasions she asked us to swear we would kill her before we let her live enfeebled. Mother was a survivor. Widowed at age 56, she moved to a Florida condominium and lived there on her own or, at times, with a man until her stroke at age 84. Her disdain for giving in to illness was evident. She had earlier refused treatment for cervical and breast cancer in situ. Despite a great deal of advice to the contrary, she declined any type of surgical treatment, stating she would rather be dead than mutilated. As things turned out she was right. She outlived both diseases. Although she had mild congestive heart failure (CHF) and hints of cognitive decline, she remained very much her own person, with strong views that she did not hesitate to share.

All that changed in May 1999, when she had a stroke. Because she had

---

This chapter will be included in the authors' forthcoming book, *It Shouldn't Be This Way: The Failure of Long-Term Care* (Vanderbilt University Press 2005).

no family or other social supports in Florida, after a brief hospitalization there we moved her to Long Island, NY, near Joan, for rehabilitation. Mother recovered an amazing amount of function through rehab, and was able to walk and perform most activities of daily living on her own. But the initial signs of memory loss and confusion she had shown prior to the stroke became central thereafter, and she had periods of confusion when she did not know where she was.

Given Mother's relatively good physical functioning and our optimism that she might continue to improve, we thought assisted living would be the best of the three options we felt we had. We dismissed home care, which Mother would have preferred, on the grounds that it would be too difficult to implement. It would have required developing a living situation from scratch, and Mother had a bad track record in sustaining relationships with helpers. If a caregiver did not show up, we would be left to scramble to find a replacement. Our professional and personal aversion to nursing homes, which entail giving up so much quality of life, and our belief that Mother didn't require that kind and amount of regimentation and care, ruled out that option. Moreover, Mother had had a very bad experience when she encouraged her own father to enter a nursing home. It left her adamant that she never wanted to enter one.

Assisted living had been rapidly developing on Long Island, and overbuilding had led to excess capacity and competition. To help us identify and rank the best facilities, Robert and his wife—a social work professor and long-term care expert—tapped into their network of professional colleagues and friends. But there was little useful information; people spoke in generalities and could provide no specific feedback. Most places seemed to be part of chains owned by a few for-profit corporations. We looked at a number of facilities in areas that would be convenient for Joan and selected one that seemed pleasant and competent. The large discount it offered on the first six months' fees, in an effort to fill its empty beds, was something of an incentive as well.

When we brought our mother to the assisted living facility—which we'll call ALFI—in June 1999, she thought she was moving to a hotel. Her confusion turned out to be quite apt. The building had originally been a motel. The new owners had created an attractive common space, with dining rooms that featured wait staff, recreation facilities including a large-screen TV for videos, and even a pool table, more often used by visitors and staff than by residents. The furnishings seemed designed to please families as much or more than residents.

Mother's room looked very much like what it had been, a fair-sized motel room, with its own bathroom and a refrigerator. Closet space was minimal for a permanent home. The room had a small terrace overlooking the grounds. She seemed contented. This was all the space she wanted, she said.

The first night was difficult. Mother became agitated and disoriented. The staff called Joan, who returned to calm her. Rather than just being a step in adjusting to new surroundings, it was the beginning of what would become a routine. During those first months, Mother called Joan several times a night. At that point she could still usually keep track of weekdays and weekends, and Joan left a notebook by Mother's bed, with her local number and the number of her weekend home. Later, the notebook would prove useful as a communication tool in which Mother's various therapists could report progress or problems.

### New Environment, New Lifestyle

Although assisted living facilities generally help residents with basic activities such as bathing, dressing, and eating, they focus far more on providing a home-like residential setting than on anything approaching skilled nursing care. The range of services available at ALFI was more suited to frail older persons who had decided that the effort required to maintain their homes was too great, but who were still quite capable of looking after themselves. A substantial proportion of the residents used canes or even walkers, but could function independently. At the time of her admission to ALFI, we believed that Mother was basically capable of living on her own as long as there were people around who could oversee her general routines and provide assistance in an emergency.

ALFI was fairly typical of assisted living facilities on Long Island, where monthly fees average $2,500 to $6,000. For that, its basic package consisted of the resident's room, with weekly cleaning service and linen change, three congregate meals daily, and a daytime recreation program of group activities, including bus trips to a nearby mall several times a week. Since Mother thought this was a hotel, she expected to have her bed made daily. Given the extra fees we were already paying for the additional supervision and assistance we expected she would require because of her stroke (looking in on her at night, helping her get to meals, assisting with dressing and using the toilet)—much of which she was not using—we persuaded the administration to provide daily bed make-up. In many facilities, personal care services are contracted out to independent home health care agencies, on-site or locally, but ALFI used its own staff for these.

Although the facility supplied linens, most residents brought their own furniture with them. With mother's emergency move from Florida, she had none of her furniture available. We rented some from the facility and bought some additional pieces.

New clothing was also essential. The uniform of the day was basically loose elastic-waist exercise pants and pullover tops, which were easy to put on and take off and, most importantly, washed well. Our fastidious mother, who had always fretted over her appearance, was now decked out in gym clothes. But although she was wearing only a limited number of very simple outfits, she still wanted to keep much of her former wardrobe. Indeed, her limited closet space became a serious problem. Moreover, the stroke had left her with enough residual weakness that her eating was messy, to say the least; one glance at her clothes after a meal revealed the entire menu. We tried to get her to use a washable gold lamé bib, but she was aware enough to know she didn't want to wear a bib, gold or not.

In these early days at ALFI, Mother moved slowly but was ambulatory, with or without a cane. We would take walks around the facility and the grounds. She could tolerate short trips. Joan would take her to the beauty parlor, and we would go out for lunch or dinner.

Generally, though, Mother went to the dining room for her meals, except for breakfast. Although the policy was that all residents should eat all meals in the dining room, Mother had never gotten up for breakfast in her life (as children we had made our own or relied on hired help). Her pattern of staying up late and sleeping late persisted at ALFI. She resisted getting up in time for breakfast; when she did, she wanted to eat in her room. Concerned about her missing a meal, the staff generally acceded and brought her a tray.

In the dining room, she was assigned to a table of six. After an initial honeymoon period she grew increasingly unhappy with that first placement. One man was verbally abusive to his wife, and another tablemate was a difficult, argumentative woman; Mother never got along with women who were as assertive and forceful as she was. After her requested transfer, her new dining companions were a mixed lot. Most were more functional, certainly more cognitively intact, although one man was actually more cognitively impaired. The women formed a fairly close group and seemed to support each other. Initially, they were very kind to Mother, who participated in their conversations, often taking her usual controversial stances. They seemed to tolerate her sloppy eating, and even reminded her where things were or helped her order from the menu. But their tolerance did not last long. Her tablemates started to complain to the staff, and suggested to Joan that Mother really needed a part-time companion to manage her eating and help her walk.

Whether she was that much weaker or simply less motivated to walk by herself, using a cane was no longer adequate, and the women and several other people suggested getting Mother a walker. Indeed, walkers seemed de rigueur in her new crowd. With assistance from ALFI and a prescription from her physician we ordered her one. Before our eyes Mother was turning into a little old lady.

Efforts to involve her in activities or to socialize beyond the dining room all failed. She confined herself, basically, to rearranging her closet and washing her underwear in her sink—the latter in part a falling back on lifelong habits and in part an attempt to hide her newly developed incontinence. Not only was Mother unable to get the laundry clean, so that Joan had to take it home and rewash it, but her habit of hanging it to dry on her terrace was not endearing her to the neighbors.

Instead of mingling or attending group programs, Mother expected Joan, who visited almost daily, to be her source of entertainment. Joan would end her school day at about four, then go directly to ALFI. Many days she would make tea in the communal kitchen and just sit and talk to Mother. Some days, she would accompany her to a session of word or memory games; that was the only way Mother could be coaxed into playing—she clearly loved having her daughter visible by her side. If it was a "good" day and she was calm and feeling reasonably content, Mother was pleasant to Joan and the other residents, and Joan could feel at peace. But on "bad" days, when Mother was agitated, hostile, and lashing out, it was difficult for Joan—who never got used to Mother's outbursts—to weather the storm.

### A "Hands-Off" Approach

Despite her CHF, Mother had few medical problems during her first months at ALFI, and used fewer services than she was entitled to. Although Medicare covered physical therapy for post-stroke rehabilitation, for example, Mother was often not cooperative or compliant, and eventually refused to participate at all. It was her emotional adjustment, her very demanding ways with the staff, and her refusal to get up and dressed in a timely way that seemed to be the most troublesome aspects of her life there.

Yet we did try to take advantage of what ALFI euphemistically called "wellness care," a limited program of oversight by a licensed practical nurse (LPN), who monitored residents' medications and performed basic health checks, such as periodic weights. Because of her CHF Mother would periodically retain fluid, so we attempted to organize daily weigh-ins, linked to a change in her diuretic medications, to detect and respond to early signs of fluid build-up. Even after we obtained physician orders outlining the steps to be taken, however, the staff was unwilling to take even that limited responsibility. To be fair, Mother was often unwilling and uncooperative about going downstairs to be weighed. She could be quite stubborn and difficult. We addressed the problem ourselves by putting a scale in her room, once she had a daytime aide.

ALFI's staff of LPNs and aides became very nervous when Mother complained of shortness of breath. Most of the time she was not ill but exhibiting symptoms of anxiety, but about six months after she entered ALFI she did experience a more serious episode. Joan and her husband took Mother to the emergency room, in what was to become the first of a series of hospitalizations related to her CHF.

After each of these hospitalizations the return to ALFI became more difficult. Initially we found that hiring an aide for a day or two helped Mother make the transition back. But as we saw, and heard reports of, her worsening mood and appetite, we thought it would be helpful to have ongoing assistance. We first hired two women, neither of them a certified nursing aide, as companions, to come in a few hours a day three times a week. Then we added an aide for Saturdays and Sundays, so Joan would not have to keep running back from her weekend home. And finally, as Mother's condition continued to deteriorate, we decided to bring someone in to get mother up and dressed for lunch, encourage her to eat, and assume much of the day-to-day responsibility for her, although Joan continued to visit nearly daily.

In some ways this proved a mixed blessing: more than needing all this help, Mother loved the extra attention, but it also seemed to make her even more dependent. She started to have panic attacks after the aide left at 7:00 p.m., and would call Joan each time; sometimes Joan was able to calm her down over the phone, but on numerous occasions she had to drive back to ALFI. We finally hired someone to come in at night as well. Mother alternately fought with her and enjoyed the idea of someone bringing her breakfast in the morning and otherwise waiting on her. But there was little else for the aide to do. She would watch Mother sleep or roam around her room, but had little effect on her outbursts or wandering. We decided to cut back and again have just the one daytime aide.

In fact, the ALFI management was at that point *insisting* that we have someone there all day. That meant, we pointed out, that at $12/hour for an aide, on top of the fees we were paying ALFI, assisted living was proving more expensive than a skilled nursing facility. This was the only way in which they would allow Mother to remain there, however. Reluctantly, we acquiesced. We did look at a nursing home designed to care for persons with dementia, but it was so institutionally drab and socially sterile that we could not envision anyone with as much cognitive function as our mother still had going there. The need for extra assistance raised again the option of her living in the community with full-time help, but the logistical complexities still seemed too great.

Although we had believed that "assisted living" would merge a comfortable environment with a minimal to moderate level of extra care, this was not the model we had bought into, we were discovering. This pattern of being pressured into hiring private aides was prevalent at ALFI; the facility's expectation was that despite families' payments for a basic set of services, outside help would be hired to actually look after residents. Clearly we were not the only family required to supplement the meager services ALFI provided; as we spent more time with the women we hired we discovered a whole community of aides and "companions," a common presence in the lobby and at activities. While they knew each other and worked together, they often had tense relationships with the ALFI staff over where the responsibilities of one group or the other started and ended.

## Bridging the Gaps

We were fortunate in finding an aide who was very reliable and responsible. But it was precisely her sense of duty and caring that brought her into conflict with staff and management. Although they had insisted we hire someone, they were angry when the aide demanded services to which Mother was entitled: in effect, we now had our own monitor overseeing what little care ALFI actually provided, and the facility did not appreciate it.

Having an all-day aide for Mother meant she was neater and cleaner, and getting more out of meals. The aide was a very positive, upbeat, warm person, who recognized the importance of Mother being socially stimulated and part of the group, even if she didn't want to be. She could often get Mother to interact more with the other residents; on good days Mother could entertain others with tales of her past exploits and conquests, including the relationships she'd had since her husband's death almost thirty years before.

At the same time, Mother still slept late most mornings and only rarely participated in activities. The aide, who was fond of playing bingo to relieve the monotony of her day, would try to engage Mother in the game, but Joan would come in to find her dozing, instead. And although her behavior was better in some ways, Mother was prone to bouts of anger, many times ordering the aide to go away. The aide could usually flatter and cajole her out of these and, if not, seemed to know when to leave the room and give her a chance to cool off, instead.

After each of these episodes Mother would revert back to a contrite, compliant, almost childlike demeanor. Although she had been a "tough cookie" with an acerbic tongue, Mother had always had the ability to charm people, too, using a flirtatious, coy manner to do so. This same dichotomy continued after her stroke, but as almost a pale imitation of her old pattern; it was even harder to watch than in the past, and Joan was frequently embarrassed. While Mother had been outspoken in the past, now she displayed a new rudeness and lack of control, loudly commenting on people's appearance and actions. The stroke had left her less inhibited, but her behavior made Joan more uptight. Nevertheless, it was a definite psychological help for us to know that Mother had someone who would advocate for her and keep her safe in Joan's absence. And however much having an aide with Mother improved the quality of her life, in many respects it was benefiting Joan's at least as much.

## Escalating Conflicts

As Mother's mental state deteriorated she began to wander outside her room at night. Often half naked, she would roam the halls in search of snacks or water, or knock on other residents' doors. One night she left the faucets running and flooded her room. She had lost all ability to monitor her behavior or recognize how inappropriate it was. In her anxiety she would also lash out, verbally and sometimes physically, at anyone in her path. Although she could show remorse afterward, she appeared not to remember her actions, and would vehemently deny them.

Her troublesome behavior warranted a psychiatric consult. We opted to use a psychiatrist who already worked with ALFI, hoping he could help them develop a behavioral approach that would minimize the use of psychoactive drugs. The staff, however, wanted assurances that Mother would be sedated enough to avert her disruptive actions. Thus began our difficult journey to find the right combination of medications that could control her yet cause neither somnolence nor an adverse reaction. There is no predetermined level for that—it requires observing the patient closely and making gradual adjustments. Not surprisingly, the staff was not up to the task. Even with prompting they were unable to organize any systematic record of observations that could guide the prescribing physician. Instead, he had to respond primarily to crises. Unfortunately, there was no shortage of those.

Once again the ALFI management called us in for a case conference, and insisted that we now have an aide with Mother every night as well as all day. After failing to convince them that there were other ways to solve the problem, we agreed to hire someone. We could appreciate that they were short-staffed, especially at night, and that Mother required more attention than they could provide, but hiring a full-time attendant seemed wasteful and extravagant. Since there were other residents with similar needs, we suggested, why not have each family pay a little more to buy, in effect, part of one person's services? Economic sense notwithstanding, ALFI did not want to foster any arrangement that would require taking any responsibility or initiative. The facility continued to require each family to hire its own workers.

### The Next Move

Mother's behavior continued to worsen. Her eating got sloppier; she wandered more. She would ramble out to the front desk, or call there to demand help. The ALFI staff claimed that other residents were complaining about her. It was impossible for her to remember directions or restrictions, even those that involved her safety. We had asked the staff to lock her terrace door but they refused, citing fire codes. Mother continued to wander outside by herself in the evenings. The final blow occurred when she fell on the terrace after dinner one night, after the aide had left and before we had reinstated a nighttime aide; she was found with a badly cut hand, requiring another debilitating trip to the ER.

At that point ALFI presented an ultimatum: we would either have to move Mother to another facility or allow ALFI to transfer her to its special care unit for persons with dementia. Even before this incident, the ALFI administration had suggested moving Mother there (where there were supposedly more staff), but we had resisted the idea: the rationale for using an assisted living facility was to preserve Mother's quality of life as long as possible. Already, on a couple of occasions, ALFI had moved Mother to this unit in the middle of the night, without letting us know, and it had been a shock for Joan to arrive for a visit and find Mother in this highly restricted setting. The individual rooms of the dementia unit were similar to those throughout ALFI, but the comfort of the regular common rooms and public areas was missing. Life was much more regimented and the setting much more spartan, with residents eating separately from the rest of the ALFI population, and rarely leaving the unit. The dementia unit was, in effect, a locked ward in the basement.

It's not always easy to know when an adjustment here and there is no longer sufficient, and when more radical change—a different kind of help—is needed. We had thought that personal aides, or a change in medication, would make life at ALFI workable for Mother. We were still resisting the idea that she had to be in a special dementia unit, with all its restrictions. Although it was clear she was deteriorating and needed more supervision, she seemed more aware of her surroundings than the residents there. At the same time, we were unhappy with the inadequate attention and care ALFI was providing in its regular unit. It was becoming increasingly clear that there was a disconnect between Mother's needs and what ALFI could provide. A complete move was seeming more and more desirable.

Coincidentally, a new assisted living facility was just opening in the same area to which Joan and her husband were moving. When we met with the administrator to discuss the feasibility of transferring Mother, she was very reassuring about their commitment and capability. Yet she really had no specific plans for how to manage someone in Mother's condition. It was quite clear her enthusiasm and confidence stemmed from a strong desire to fill the facility. This time we understood, as we had not before, that empty beds can produce empty promises.

### Denouement

We finally decided to transfer Mother to another assisted living facility closer to Joan's new home, one run by a corporation that prided itself on handling "difficult" patients. This facility's dementia unit, to which Mother was admitted, was superior to ALFI's in terms of décor and a sense of openness, and had a staff that seemed more oriented to caring for persons with dementia. But although we worked hard to establish a strong relationship with staff there, Mother's condition continued to decline. She spent nine months there, hating, in her lucid moments, being with "crazy people."

Ultimately, she became frailer and required still more physical assistance and staff oversight, and we placed her in a nursing home. There, her medical and nursing care was much better coordinated, and all of it could be provided on site. No complicated transportation arrangements needed to be organized. During her last three months in the home, including her terminal illness, she never went to the hospital. Logistically, it was certainly easier for us, but not necessarily a happier experience for Mother herself. She died three months later, in May 2002.

For all of us, each step of this journey became more difficult to take. Nothing of this experience reflected the way Mother had wanted her life to end, or what we wanted for her. Despite advocating the empowerment of older persons we wound up making all the decisions, even when they clearly violated Mother's wishes. She wanted to live on her own—or, more accurately, with 24-hour assistance—in an apartment. We felt that such an arrangement was too tenuous, difficult, costly, and, ultimately, risky. In truth, though, it seems unlikely that Mother could have made better choices herself. Any option would have presented its own set of problems. It may be that the people who do best with life transitions like these are those who are more passive, flexible, and accommodating. With her strong opinions and personality, Mother was none of those.

While Mother's last days were spent as she had dreaded, Joan found herself unable ever to do enough for her, and miserable watching her decline. Robert was frustrated with his inability to create a workable solution, one that would translate into reality all the theories about how different types of care are supposed to respond to changing needs. Throughout this whole depressing time we kept thinking that if this was what *we* were experiencing, how much worse it must be for those who are totally uninformed and ill prepared. With all our knowledge, and all the support on which we could call, perhaps we underestimated the extent of one-on-one management that Mother needed. And perhaps it is just such clear vision that is critical to easing the way for both care recipient and caregiver.

We began this adventure with a strong belief that assisted living could actually fill a large part of the role nursing homes have played. We ended it much less confident that this overlap is as large as it might be. We fought hard to keep Mother in assisted living for as long as possible. Our tolerance of its limitations was greater, certainly, than the ALFI staff's. The second facility made active efforts to accommodate our mother, largely because (as we always suspected and later learned) they were under great pressure from their corporate president, a colleague with whom my wife had spoken, to do so. Left to their own devices, they too would have pressed for an earlier discharge. Although another colleague who operates a national chain of assisted living facilities regularly argues that they should be capable of handling clients like our mother, it is unlikely that we could have found another assisted living facility in the same area that would have accepted her.

If there are second thoughts about this experience, they are probably that we did not buy enough additional hours of aides' time. Despite economics and a sense of fairness about what an assisted living facility should provide, we could have bought more personal care for Mother and perhaps enabled her to remain in an assisted living environment until she died. It would have been extravagant but it was possible. We will never know how it might have affected the quality of her last three months.

Our experience suggests that our society needs to create a hybrid between assisted living and nursing homes, facilities that can provide more care than the former in a more livable environment than the latter. It should not be necessary to choose one or the other. The additional care might be paid for in increments, as a person's status deteriorates. Since one of us is a teacher, this seems analogous to the case of the special education student whose needs cannot be met in a regular classroom. There is a mandate to find "the least restrictive environment" in which to educate a special needs child. Our mother was like that child, in that the traditional settings and protocols did not really meet her needs. The educational model emphasizes inclusion wherever possible, through the provision of additional aides and services. The health care system could learn from this model and have the additional personnel it needs on site. Otherwise, just as children fall through the cracks and are lost, so too will frail and needy older persons and their family caregivers.

# 6  Family Caregiving: Both Sides Now

*Jane Bendetson*

## I. The Solace of a Sonnet, the Sanctuary of the Classroom

My husband had his first heart attack when our son, Eric, was seven. With that event, chronic illness became omnipresent and omnipotent in our family's life. I was terrified. Life was so fragile and our family so threatened. I feared that at any point I could become solely responsible for providing a reliable income. Gone were the halcyon days of stay-at-home mommy, lady who lunched, writer who fantasized about the Great American Novel. In due course my husband returned to work, but the potential pressure for me to support the family was ever present.

I learned that a highly prestigious prep school in Manhattan had an opening in the Upper School English department. Although I had never taught, except as a graduate assistant, I managed to become an instant English teacher. The salary was low but it was a steady job, and my holidays would correspond with Eric's.

So began 23 years of trying to balance the priorities of being virtually a single mother, a caregiver, a writer from 5:00 a.m. to 6:30 a.m., and a teacher spending exhausted hours on preparation in an effort to be as indispensable as possible. I pretended everything was fine, desperately trying to create a "normal family life," whatever that may be, and, of course, failing, for chronic illness is a family affair. I joyfully went to Eric's basketball games and tennis matches but hospital corridors became a familiar labyrinth. With each heart attack my husband's physical abilities diminished, and the ticking continuum of his anger toward the "well" world would erupt and then subside into the lethargy of depression.

---

Part I of this chapter is adapted from Jane Bendetson's contribution to the first edition of *Always on Call*.

My world became ever more compartmentalized as I vainly hoped to lock heart disease into a small cubbyhole of my life. As it became impossible for my husband to attend social functions, I went alone—married, yet single. One concert, dance, opera subscription after another was canceled. As his world became ever smaller, so did mine. Yet I could not afford to allow, nor did I want, his illness to intrude on my school life. Also, I was afraid lest I ever be vulnerable, less than conscientious, or less than in total command of the material. If I were fired, downsized, what would we do? The question haunted, always.

Although Eric became more independent, my husband became ever more dependent. I took over all money matters, all decisions, all planning. Every pill, 17 a day at one point, had to be put out each morning. The turning, lifting, and moving, the caring for rashes, hives, and sores were daily responsibilities. No aide could ever cook properly for his special diets, so I made separate dinners for him and Eric. As I had so little control over my personal life, the classroom became a world wherein the structure of a sonnet gave solace and the ambiguity in poetry resonated with my own.

Collegiality was limited to being given a lighted cigarette, even though my co-workers knew I had quit smoking, when between classes I was told that my husband was being rushed to the hospital less than a year after the first attack. I quickly learned that chronic illness is embarrassing, boring, and frightening to people, almost as if it were a communicable disease. Consequently, associates kept their distance. I also wanted a life of my own, not defined by my husband's illness, so when someone did ask how he was, I'd smile and say, "Fine." It's not that they really wanted to know, and I needed to keep the door to that cubbyhole firmly closed. No one, of course, ever asked how I was doing or coping.

The school administrators, if aware of my situation at all, didn't acknowledge it. They indifferently rejected my occasional request during emergencies for a few extra days to write reports, or a day off, so I stopped asking. Even after an all-night stay in the emergency room or outside the ICU, I would be in class at 8:30 a.m. to teach *Paradise Lost*.

At first it had been a job, a paycheck, then a need, and finally salvation. It took me a long time to realize that the depth of the need to be *me*, not "the wife," the unseen caregiver, was so great that I endured humiliation, genteel cruelty, and indifference I would never accept today. I leached the vitality of the students, buoyed by their energy. The intensity of adolescent angst mollified my own. There was triumph and laughter. Days had structure and the year a nine-month gestation, a world of 50-minute hours rather than one in which a lifetime disappeared in a moment.

When I moved to another prestigious high school and became the token female in the English Department, the chairman began the first departmental meeting by saying, "Gentlemen and Jane . . ." and then suggested that I knit the gentlemen departmental ties. I bridled but said nothing. I was new and a working woman/mother/caregiver. I couldn't jeopardize my position by reacting negatively.

Once, after a particularly grueling crisis, through which I had met every class and every appointment, I asked the dean if I could be excused from an in-service program because I was truly exhausted. He denied my request. It was only the kids who asked if I was ill, because I looked so tired.

Several years after that, however, when I was scheduled to teach a late afternoon class in the winter, I went to the same dean and told him that my husband had just been discharged from the hospital after a two-month stay. Although an aide was with him, I explained, my husband's depression came not on "little cat feet" but on thundering hooves when the sun went down. If I were home, I could alleviate his misery somewhat with chitchat and tales from the world outside. I asked if I could please change schedules with another teacher. At first he refused but then, on second thought, because it was for the benefit of my husband, the patient, he assented.

There were many indignities over the years, when I was given heavier teaching loads than others, onerous extra duties, but never the privilege of missing a faculty meeting to get to the hospital. Perhaps the administration realized I couldn't refuse. Everything crystallized when my husband died at home on a Thanksgiving Day. On Friday, I phoned the head of my department and said, "My husband died yesterday."

"What am I supposed to do about that?"

"I'd like a week off and thought you might need time to find a substitute."

"I don't know if I can do that."

"I'll tell the person just where each class is in its work. I really need a week."

Finally, he reluctantly granted me the time.

I planned with infinite care what I would say to the students when I returned, knowing that they would have learned about my husband's death during my absence. I felt that what I said that day would be more important than anything I had ever taught, because possibly they could learn to see mortality without fear. They were terrific and responded as I hoped, no longer uncertain about how to behave about his death, or how to relate to me, a new widow. I told them how my godson nursed lustily at breakfast the week before, adding that leaving life is as natural as coming into it. After assuring them I was still the same person, we went on to discuss John Donne's "Holy Sonnets." So as I went to lunch, I really thought things were going to be all right.

On the way I met the headmaster who said, "I hope you have a good estate lawyer so everything can be settled without your missing any school."

"He's very good. There will be no problem."

I didn't go to lunch. I went back to the classroom, my sanctuary.

## II. Broken Vessels, Broken Promise

That terrifying day of his father's first heart attack, I somehow had to explain to seven-year-old Eric that everything would be "fine," although Daddy would be in the hospital for a long time. Planning carefully, I prepared his favorite dish, lamb chops. Just the two of us together in the kitchen, I tried to reassure him. He somehow knew this was a different "sick," suddenly leapt off his chair, came to me, put out his greasy hand, and shook my own. "We're in this alone, together."

And so we were for 23 years, 23 years of juggling demanding, conflicting roles. In all that time I was angry, lonely, frustrated, exhausted. I swore that Eric would never again be a caregiver.

### The Power of a Mantra

On August 4, 2001, I broke my promise to Eric: I became a patient and he became a caregiver. I had a stroke, a brain-injuring event that killed a significant part of the left side of my brain.

The course of cardiac disease or stroke can't be predicted. My husband knew that a heart attack at any moment could be the final one, and now I, too, know another stroke can kill me. Sirens and monitors punctuated the rhythm of my husband's heartbeats; for me, it is silent images on a CAT scan.

That day, I'd planned to finish writing an article about a local road race, and to celebrate the summer with houseguests. Early that morning, Eric, Lisa (my beloved daughter-in-law), Chou Chou (my companion dog), and I started out to watch this special event. My stroke, however, intervened. After the week in the hospital that followed, the article was never written.

Throughout our earlier life in caregiving, Eric felt I'd been a dynamo, so energetic, invincible. Suddenly, I'd fallen curled up by the road. He was terrified, hovered constantly in the hospital while Lisa bolstered him. When he realized I wasn't going to die, his humor returned. But Eric and Lisa both knew well some of the problems of caregivers. When they were children both had to help their mothers; both their childhoods were shortened and shriveled.

In the emergency room, I obsessively babbled about going home for the expected guests. Constantly, I chanted my mantra. "I'm fine. Nothing's wrong with me." That's what I felt. Without paralysis or any other physical change, I marched down the halls of the hospital and thought therapists were ridiculous when they asked me, "Can you walk up the stairs?" What a stupid question. "I'm fine."

When, toward the end of the week, Eric and my doctor suggested moving me to the rehabilitation hospital, I shrieked as if I were in a Greek tragedy. I had to have quiet, I said, not be in a noisy hospital. Reading, writing, finishing that article would be impossible in a hospital. I won and went home. In retrospect, a different choice may well have been better.

Although Eric and Lisa were relieved to be bringing me home, they were uncertain about what would happen next. He gently asked if it might be a good idea to stay with me that first night. "Oh! Fine." Nothing else mattered except being home with Chou Chou, ocean, and horizon.

## The Vampire, Coffee, and Other Imponderables

Experienced with taking care of his father, having worked as a clinical social worker and a lawyer, Eric wanted to have full-time caregivers in my home although I was mobile. How silly! I demanded to be alone, to write, to read. Eric arranged for visiting nurses and others to come instead.

My life centered around words, but this was the first time I heard the word "aphasia." Many people explained the definition, but it was meaningless to me. Since my stroke, I've learned the meaning within my being, within my soul. Aphasia describes an acquired disability characterized by an impairment of speaking, listening, reading, writing, and, most of all, comprehending. But I didn't know I was aphasic and, naturally, assumed others understood what I said. Soon, however, I thought they were using a different language. I had lost communication. Words were imprisoned, tangled in a web. Now I wonder how the people coming into my house then figured out my garbled words.

A young man whom I called "Vampire," an epithet he enjoyed, arrived daily to take blood tests. A speech therapist came in twice a week for a few weeks. The poor young woman must have been overwhelmed by my arrogance in displaying my English skills. I didn't need her. In addition, non-professional caregivers, a cleaning woman and a gardener who knew me well, watched over me.

Every so often a supervisor nurse dropped in, but one time a different woman arrived and sat down in the living room. Officious and condescending, with clipboard and pen, she asked inane questions.

Finally she added, "How about a cup of coffee?"

Ah! At last, something sensible, I felt. I jumped up to go to the kitchen, put water in the kettle, and got beans from the freezer. "This coffee is special; African coffee has more caffeine." Pshaw. Of course, she'd want cream. I said, "I always drink coffee black and, certainly, without a grain of sugar to ruin the flavor." She nodded and wrote. I ground the beans, carefully counting aloud one to twenty, plus four more pulses. I smiled. "I have no idea why I count like that. Maybe tradition." She nodded patronizingly, once again scribbling on the clipboard.

I gave her the cup of my ambrosia. "Oh, I don't want any," she said.

Now this, I thought, is really the most unbelievable stupidity.

After what seemed like forever she smiled, glanced at the clipboard, said, "You're living here well. You're fine."

"Well, of course I'm fine." Finally she left. Why do people think I'm dumb?

Later, someone told me the woman was an occupational therapist. I had no idea what an occupational therapist did, but I knew she didn't like my coffee.

But the Vampire listened to what I said. One day, I talked about poets and poetry between World Wars I and II. I went on and on for quite a while. When he was leaving, he turned to me and said, "You spoke each word, every syllable without a problem and your mind is perfectly clear. You're going to be fine." Strange. I never imagined I wasn't fine in any way. I remembered his words, though, and was comforted. But Eric and Lisa were my salvation.

## My Son the Caregiver

When I was being discharged from the hospital, I had ignored the doctor's unpleasant, emphatic instructions. At home, however, I had to absorb the changes in my life: no alcohol, not even a glass of wine at dinner; no caffeine except one cup of coffee a day. Disaster, even though people said,

"Decaf tastes the same." Nonsense! Then more insanity: I couldn't go beyond the yard—couldn't drive, couldn't go over the fence at the bottom of the backyard to walk on the beach, couldn't even walk along the roads or in the woods. In addition, Eric, my "attorney of power," was in charge of my money. I had always been independent but now I was a dependent. Horror! I had no freedom. I had no control. Eruption. Rage. After all, I'm fine.

When my New York friends phoned almost daily, I told them melodramatically I was manacled and abused. Immediately, they called Eric. He and Lisa arrived in a fury. They exclaimed they were trying to help me any way they could, but never, ever wanted to hurt me. I saw reflections of caregiving, generation by generation. Humbly, abashed, I apologized profusely. Long ago, as a caregiver, I appreciated the thanks, apologies, even a flower after all the demands of my patient. Now, I pleaded with my primary caregivers to see *me*, a person, more than a patient or object. Ironic: as a caregiver I'd felt invisible; this time, as a patient, I also felt unseen.

During our talk, we calmed down and planned a schedule, which had to be flexible, considering their work. Of course, I would call them in an emergency. I looked forward to Mondays when Eric would come to write checks and take care of other chores. Before the stroke he was never concerned about money. Now he had to be responsible. On Thursdays, Lisa squeezed time into her practicing lawyer schedule, so she could call me for my market list and bring groceries to me.

I wondered how Eric felt about these tasks and about having to drive me to doctor appointments. I felt guilty about being such a burden but was glad that, at least, they didn't have to live with me, didn't have to be in the same home with chronic illness. Meanwhile, I was comforted that they were only half an hour away. I never wanted them ever to feel guilty about anything while being caregivers. I remembered how even though I had tried so hard not to feel guilty, I had, simply because I was healthy. There are so many aspects of caregiving.

When I had to absorb changes to live, Eric, too, had to accept new ways. He had to become a rock, too solid, too fast. Certainly I could no longer be the stable one. Also, although he's never said it, I knew he was disappointed and frustrated that I was not a wordsmith any more. In addition, he couldn't help in any way to return my lost fluency.

I remember when I had Eric read something I'd just written.

"Is it funny?" I asked.

"Yes, it's funny, very funny." A long moment and then, "Mums, you're so much better than this. Please don't publish it."

A pang. "Well, you know, I always rewrite." Later I reread it, knew it needed a bit of work, but Eric had said it was funny. For some reason, though, I never sent it to the editor.

One day, I heard a knock at the front door, opened it, and looked up into the face of an adolescent boy at least ten feet tall.

"Hi. I'm on the high school team." I had figured that without much effort. "We're trying to get money for a trip to work out before the season. Here are my credentials to collect."

"I'd help, but have no money."

"That's all right. I can take a check for the high school."

"I have no check."

He looked at me sympathetically. "Oh. That's all right. I understand." He left.

He didn't understand at all. I closed the door, guffawed. What a sweet kid. Of course, I'm fine.

## Accepting the Reality

After all, nothing's wrong with me. I "read" the *New York Times* each morning and muttered, "Ambiguous." Thought, "Why are these writers working this way? They always used to do better." I read a sentence and then a paragraph over and over. I realized I wasn't reading well. At last, it crept up on me, slipped from "I'm fine" to "I'm not fine." I'm so gratified my mantra had protected me from the devastating pain all that time. Syllable by syllable my barricades crumbled and I drowned.

Eric and Lisa tried to buoy me. One evening he phoned me: "Mums, we thought the three of us would go to dinner. Very casual."

"Wonderful. I'd like that."

At the restaurant, so many people, I laughed. "Think it's so crowded and I'm a New Yorker."

The waiter wanted the orders. I, the garrulous, gregarious person was silent. I pathetically looked to Eric, cowered, unable to say anything. He told me how saddened he was seeing me like that. Where was his mother?

The Vampire and other professional caregivers were gone. Silence. I couldn't connect with anyone. I mangled my words. If I could only be a hermit, I'd be fine. I knew my mind was clear, although others didn't understand what I was saying. Eric and Lisa could understand what I said but they couldn't be quite sure how much I understood them. I talked and hugged my dog, who attentively listened. I felt conversation with the wind and the surf, the birds and rain. The language of Beethoven, of Bach, sang to me.

What I loved so much was gone, truly gone. I clicked on the computer. Don't quit; try slowly to read what I've written. Jumbled hieroglyphs, no words, no sentences. Above all, I was scared, but I hoped. "Haven't really worked on anything for a long time. Just practice. Everything will be exactly as it was." I dutifully turned on the machine each day, clacked away every day to write in my old journal. "Go on, get those fingers moving, the mind busy." I'd print out and put every page into a drawer, never read them for months. I thought all that practice would make everything fine. My words, my sentences, even paragraphs would be there. Finally, I read my last entry. Nothing. Empty. Silent. Forever.

Close friends would visit, smile, talk. I'd instantly take up my clown mask, "chat," make coffee. Many people had said, "I'm in awe the way you just go on. No wonder that you're cheerful. You're healing."

I'd smile. "Thanks." From the depth of the abyss they'd never hear a whisper or a distant echo.

Only Eric heard the reverberation. In desperation, he suggested stroke support groups, senior exercise classes, yoga, books I could read, gardening, a needlework club, knitting, even watching TV. Nothing.

Keening. What to do? Everything gone. Once upon a time . . . Fetally curled. Why go on? There was one option for me. Why not? Use it. I stared day by day, night by night, into infinity, eternity.

In fall, a gardener friend dropped by. "I've got these bulbs, marvelous colors. Look."

How could these dull, brown bulbs possibly bloom gloriously? I morosely contemplated that maybe I'd not be here in spring, and imagined people would say, "How wonderful. She loved her garden so much." So I asked my friend, "Where do you think people will see the tulips best?"

"I think it'd be better to put them in a place where you would see them."

"Oh?" I paused. "OK." Found a spot. Dug one bulb and another with the sun warming my back. A worm. I carefully put it way deep in the soil. The robins would arrive again and could eat the poor thing. Give it a good warm home. Ridiculous, but it made me feel good.

Across the yard, low tide brought the aroma of seaweed and water creatures. Many people dislike the pungency, but that sea fragrance is cologne for me. At the fence, my dog and I gazed as the water lapped the rocks. I hugged my funny dog and told her, "We'll go down. Promise." Tail wagged, mouth opened, panted, tongue curled. "Look at all the tidal pools with treasures." I wondered if other treasures were cradling in the garden as if in tidal pools. "Chou Chou, let's see what we can find."

> To see a World in a grain of sand,
> And a Heaven in a wild flower,
> Hold infinity in the palm of your hand,
> And Eternity in an hour.

As a child, I memorized that quatrain. Always have liked William Blake; hoped to find a new way in those lines. I lived with T. S. Eliot's "Waste Land" and "Hollow Men," but now I'm also able to see Blake's "grain of sand" and "wild flower."

## Reconnecting with Words

At last I was humbled, willing to meet with a speech-language pathologist. After a long wait for an appointment, Eric drove me to the rehabilitation hospital. The therapist, Eric, and I chatted. The therapist, Dr. Steven Belanger, asked what he could do to help.

I said, "Here and there I know words but I can't remember them, can't say them. I spell and even speak esoteric words but I can't get simple, one-syllable ones."

Dr. Belanger nodded. "I think we can do some things. You should come three times a week."

A squeak: "Three times a week? So much time? I have so much to do, garden and things—something."

But I was excited. People had tried to help, but I felt at last that someone who understood would work with me.

So I went to my therapist's office, three times a week, and we worked. Eric would phone after each session. Just hearing my voice, he knew I was happy, doing well.

In the first days we talked about various things and did many tests. Soon Dr. Belanger said, "Someone mentioned you had wanted to write."

"Yes," I said, "but probably it won't work."

"Shall we try?"

"I dunno." I was afraid it wouldn't help. The idea of trying was incredibly more terrifying than facing a blank page of paper used to be. "Maybe, I guess."

"May I see a couple of things you wrote before and after the stroke?"

At the next session I brought in a few pages, looked out a window feeling like a student bringing an assignment. He finished the pages, said, "I hope you go on. You should. You write so well."

For the first time in months, I felt maybe . . . maybe. He actually complimented me, supported me.

We worked and worked. He told me that writing was one of the most sophisticated skills to conquer in aphasia. Oh, how well I know. The results were only inky fingers from an old, leaky pen. I said, "Maybe quit. I've tried and tried, really with no effect. It's frustrating."

"I know you've worked hard. You're tired, discouraged, frustrated. I can understand if you don't want to go on." He waited. I was quiet. My mentor then explained how little literature there is on improving writing in aphasic individuals.

"You mean, if I can be a guinea pig for research, then I won't have to feel guilty."

"Perhaps." He grinned, then gave me a couple of articles from the *Times*, from 1992. "These are the only ones I've found for the general reader about aphasia. You may be interested in them."

Such a privilege to read when other patients can't.

At our next session I announced, "I've never accepted that I have a disability. Amazing. I don't feel disabled. When I see those who work here, for months, to say even one word, the name of a loved one, I'm so thankful. I want to write for all those who are silent, who truly don't have voices, words." Banging on the table I vowed, "I'm going to do it."

On and on we went, trying one way after another, and he'd constantly nag me about grammar, grammar. It was back to basics. Beginning once more.

I'll never know how this master teacher taught me, but I really learned. In a miracle, I soon wrote simple sentences that made sense.

Eric read, said, "Better," encouraged both of us. But we remember all I've lost and together we slowly acknowledge who I am now.

I struggle along word by word but there are so many other things for me to learn. There are no lamb chops, no seven-year-old little boy. Eric and I were caregivers for 23 years. Now this time I'm the patient, knowing the two sides of chronic illness. I hope wisdom will guide me ahead with the joy of each dawn, as the horizon quickens and the sky shimmers over the sea.

# 7     Bringing Up Alex: A Parent Becomes an Advocate

*Kathryn Cooper Corley*

It was late November, but I don't really remember the weather outside or the details about the trip to the hospital or what I was wearing. What I do remember is the moment he was born, my second child, and the wonder and awe that I once again felt. There was my beautiful baby boy, all eight pounds, five ounces of him! Ruddy, round faced, and crying vigorously. I remember hearing the nurse predict, commenting on the strength of his sucking reflex, that he would be a "great nurser." I remember looking across the room to my husband Jack and my mother, watching as Alex was washed, warmed, and wrapped in a blanket. I remember the feeling of immense relief that he was here and he was healthy. I remember holding him as my daughter met her new brother. I remember feeling that our family was somehow more complete.

Alex was born just before Thanksgiving. By Christmas, I knew something was wrong. My valiant attempts to nurse him had failed, and he was only slightly more receptive to bottle feedings. He gulped and gasped and choked, and took in less than half the volume of formula considered adequate. He spit up large volumes after every feeding. He never seemed to feel hunger and would sleep through the night or longer without waking for a bottle. He was not growing as expected.

I began to schedule extra appointments at the pediatrician's office to discuss my worries. The nurse patted my hand each time and assured me that babies know what they need; he would not starve himself. When his volume of formula intake began to drop from its already inadequate levels, she informed me that I worried too much and that it wasn't good for me or for the baby. One day, I called overwhelmed with worry because Alex had taken in less than six ounces of formula in the preceding 24 hours. I wanted to talk with the pediatrician. The nurse refused, reminding me that I had been told that I could use their scale to weigh Alex if I was worried, but that the doctor had other children to see—children who were "really" sick. After this rebuke, I cried and worried that maybe I was losing my mind. I called friends and family to rebuild my confidence so I could march into the doctor's office to use that scale. When the nurse realized that Alex had lost nearly a pound in less than two weeks, she told me, with lowered eyes, that she would work us into the doctor's schedule.

## Labeling Alex

And so we entered life with a chronically ill child. Alex received his first label: "Failure to thrive." I cannot imagine a worse insult to a mother's heart than to describe her child as "failing to thrive." Of course, plenty of other labels have since been applied. Alex is six years old now and, in the strictest sense, I suppose he could still be considered a "failure to thrive." He is extremely small for his age, falling below the second percentile in height. After an arduous quest, he was finally diagnosed with a rare neuromuscular metabolic disorder, mitochondrial encephalomyopathy, considered to be progressive and terminal. As a result, he has a seizure disorder, an irregular electrocardiogram indicative of hypertrophic cardiomyopathy, poor muscle tone, and neuropathy. His gastrointestinal tract works very poorly. His acid reflux was severe enough to warrant surgical intervention at age two. He takes more than 90 percent of his nutrition via gastrostomy tube. His fasting intolerance and resulting hypoglycemia necessitate multiple tube feedings, boosted with cornstarch, during the day and continuous alimentation via feeding pump at night. He is fed a highly specialized formula that we adapt further to meet his metabolic needs by adding a prescribed course of coenzyme Q10, carnitine, vitamins, and antioxidants, which may slow down the progression of the disease.

Alex experienced a strokelike event when he was two that left him with weakness on his left side, speech problems, and difficulty in retrieving and using words he knows, though his comprehension of language was left intact. Alex fatigues easily so he requires frequent rest periods and extra sleep at night.

Yet none of these descriptions captures Alex's spirit. He most certainly is thriving beyond what I had dared think possible. His laughter is buoyant and infectious. He is gentle, kind, and loving, and makes friends easily. He loves trains and cars, painting at his easel, riding his bicycle, playing soccer, and going to school. We walk to a neighborhood preschool together three mornings each week. It is an inclusive setting with typically developing children. His teacher told me recently that she has largely forgotten there is anything special about Alex—the most wonderful thing she could have said!

## The Extraordinary Becomes Routine

But *we* haven't forgotten. Alex's care consumes far more time than that required for a typically developing child. Shortly after Alex's birth, we began to accumulate extra people in our lives: first a feeding therapist, a pediatric neurologist, a pediatric gastroenterologist, and a physical therapist, then many more to follow. With each new professional, we added appointments and homework. Everyone wanted to see him at least monthly when he was an infant. The therapists recommended sessions once or twice a week. The pediatrician and gastroenterologist wanted to weigh him weekly. We shuttled to and from four to five appointments outside our home each week.

At home, we stretched Alex's tight muscles and his neck, and we encouraged him to use his weak muscles each day as instructed by the physical therapist. The feeding therapist felt that Alex was "neurologically disorganized" at feeding times, and recommended special techniques to reduce outside stimulation. First we massaged and "brushed" him, then lay him on his side in a dark, quiet room, turning his face toward a blank wall, applying gentle pressure with our fingers to the sides of his face to help strengthen his sucking. I wasn't even allowed to look my precious child in the eyes and sing to him while I fed him, because it made it too hard for him to concentrate on eating. The whole process took a little over an hour, and we fed him every three hours, continuing throughout the night. He was on a number of medications, each with its own schedule and recommended protocol. Between feeding and medicating and stretching and positioning and encouraging Alex to move, transporting him to and from medical appointments and therapy, our lives were completely consumed. Neither Jack nor I was getting adequate sleep—at most three to four hours of broken sleep a night for months at a time.

Before Alex was born, our daughter, Sarah, was the center of our universe. After his birth, she seemed to fade from my daily life because of the time that feeding Alex required. She spent hours in waiting rooms at doctors' offices, sitting on the sidelines as Alex received therapy, shuttling between grandparents and neighbors as we traveled out of town to meet with new doctors. In short, Sarah's position shifted. Though we purposefully carved out time especially for her, she still became the *other* child—the "well sibling."

At home, Sarah was angelic during that time. At five years of age, she seemed to sense how precarious the situation was. At school, however, her teacher began to notice periods when Sarah seemed unable to focus; she wondered whether Sarah might have attention-deficit disorder. We consulted with a psychologist, who concluded that it was the stress of living with a very sick sibling that was interfering with Sarah's ability to concentrate at school. Amazing... *I* certainly was having difficulty concentrating. How could I fail to realize that Sarah might have the same problem? All of us were affected by this change in our lives. The impact was huge.

For one, my career goals changed substantially. Although I'd worked hard to obtain my master's degree, I was no longer able to keep up with the demands of a full-time career. I had been working for a family-friendly organization with flexible scheduling options and on-site childcare, but after Alex's birth I needed to scale back first to part-time and then even further to working from home. Eventually, it became clear that I could not continue to meet both Alex's and my employer's needs successfully.

Changes in my career meant changes in our family's financial status. Despite our misgivings about how we would survive on one salary, I resigned from my job—a loss of more than 40 percent of our income, just when our medical expenses were increasing more than we could have imagined. We chewed through our hard-earned savings and started racking up debt. Eventually, as Alex's health stabilized and he began attending school, I began a part-time consulting job that I could do from home, with hours and terms flexible enough to leave time for therapy sessions and medical appointments.

The workload associated with Alex's medical problems also put great strain on my marriage, initially. Jack and I had too little time to spend with one another, we were chronically tired, and we were constantly struggling to renegotiate and redefine roles to meet everybody's needs. There just wasn't enough time to concentrate on our relationship. We tried on several occasions to schedule a weekend getaway for just the two of us, but each time a medical crisis occurred and the trip had to be cancelled. Fortunately, we have survived the hardest of times and have learned to work together as a team rather than to pull apart.

## New Roles, New Priorities

There are literally hundreds of incidents I can cite related to Alex's condition and its impact on us. But several stand out as marking significant changes in our relationship with the legion of professionals who were now part of our lives.

One day Sarah watched as I held Alex during a "grand mal" or generalized tonic-clonic seizure. My husband was on the phone making plans with his father for a sorely needed beach vacation for the entire extended family. He hung up and called 911. A fire truck arrived first, then a police car, and finally the ambulance. Alex was no longer convulsing; he was breathing, but non-responsive. The EMTs asked me if this was his normal state. They gave my daughter a teddy bear, I think. All our neighbors were gathering in their yards, and one said she would take Sarah to McDonald's.

Only one of us could ride in the ambulance with Alex—I already knew that from an earlier emergency. I climbed in without even giving Jack the option. We arrived at the hospital, where the emergency-room staff told me that Alex had had a seizure (as if I didn't know that!) and that any testing just then was not likely to show us anything new. (Understand that many, many tests had been performed in the previous months, all with seemingly normal results.)

After we were discharged from the emergency room I sat in the pediatrician's office, feeling totally wrung out. Once again, none of the doctors seemed to have any idea of what might be causing Alex's symptoms. Passing in the hallway, Alex's pediatrician saw me still sitting there after I was supposed to have left. She gently approached and sat close to me, put her hand on mine, and told me how much she wished she could make this better. She had run out of ideas, she confessed, and had shared Alex's case with all the doctors in her practice, and others. In fact, there was a steak dinner in it for anyone who could help her identify the cause of Alex's symptoms. Diagnosing a difficult case like this one required collecting clues, she explained, and that took time.

That discussion helped me realize that I, too, had an important role to play among all the professionals: collecting those clues. I was with Alex almost every hour of the day. I knew him better than anyone else. I also realized that each of Alex's doctors had responsibility for hundreds of children, while I had responsibility only for my own. No matter how wonderful or motivated the doctors were to find answers and solutions, no one was more motivated than I. He was my baby.

I was also to learn there would be times when I'd have to be more as-sertive with the health care team. When Alex was about 16 months old his growth seemed to stall completely, and then he began losing weight. We made the difficult decision to provide him with supplemental feed-ings by nasojejunal tube. I understood that this tube would enter his nose, run down his esophagus, through his stomach, and into his small intes-tine. We would hook the tubing up to a feeding pump at night and deliver formula to supplement the tiny amount of food and formula he ate and drank during the day. The tubing would be inserted in the radiology de-partment so the doctor could see its location as it snaked through Alex's GI tract.

Only one parent was allowed to remain with Alex, terrified though he was. He was old enough to put up a fight, but too young to understand what was happening to him. We requested a sedative to help calm him and were told that it wasn't necessary. But Alex wouldn't hold still. He screamed in fear. His nose began to bleed as the doctor jabbed the tubing in over and over. Alex was placed on his back on a table. His hands and arms were tied above his head with a blanket, and his legs were wrapped as well. Three radiology technicians, complete strangers to Alex, helped hold him down.

Alex yelled for help, for me, for his father. He couldn't fathom why we wouldn't come to his aid. Just as it seemed that the tubing was positioned properly, Alex would manage to jerk himself enough to dislodge it. The process would start over. It seemed to take forever. I stood outside the door—Jack was in there with him—listening to his screams, feeling help-less, and crying for him.

I don't know why I didn't storm in and insist that they stop. I suppose that I knew that the feeding tube was necessary, and since I had never experienced this before I thought that they knew best. Later I learned that the protocol varies. Some facilities sedate children for such procedures, but because it takes more time to wait for the sedative to work than to run the tubing, some doctors prefer to press ahead without sedation.

I vowed, at that moment, that Alex's fear and pain would be taken se-riously, and that ministering to his spirit would always take priority over saving time.

## Searching for a Diagnosis

It was nearly three years before Alex received a diagnosis. His symptoms were so scary: terrible feeding problems, failure to thrive, chronic vomiting and diarrhea, seizures. He looked awful. Nearly all of the many tests and diagnostic procedures came back within normal limits. The nurses would call with the "good news" that everything looked fine. It was not good news to me. It meant that we still didn't know. I sometimes felt blamed for Alex's condition, because *why* he was experiencing his difficulties was so unclear. With the addition of every new professional, I felt my parenting skills being placed under further scrutiny, far beyond what parents of typical children experience.

Without a diagnosis, we had no idea what the prognosis was, and I frequently wondered whether Alex would live to his next birthday. I wanted to be extremely aggressive in finding answers for him, but I felt I was walking a tightrope, balancing the weighty responsibility of ensuring that Alex got adequate assessment with the equally weighty fear of alienating all the medical professionals upon whom I felt my child's life depended! Because his doctors were unsure what was going on, treatment options were limited. We spent a tremendous amount of time and energy on strategies that didn't work or were, in retrospect, completely inappropriate, simply because we didn't yet have a name for his disorder. I was frustrated because it seemed to me that too much time passed between determining that a strategy was ineffective and devising a new one.

When the doctors ran out of ideas, I felt angry at what I perceived as inattention. I was desperate to find out why all of this was happening. Mostly, I just wanted someone to wave a magic wand and make it stop. I wanted to sing to Alex and look deep into his eyes while I fed him. I wanted to take him to the park instead of therapy. I wanted a good night's sleep. I wanted to shower without worrying about what was happening on the other side of the curtain. I wanted to spend time with my husband and daughter. I wanted life to be normal.

Fortunately, we received information about desperately needed community services very early on. When Alex was four months old, his feeding therapist noted that his muscle tone seemed irregular and encouraged us to seek a physical therapy evaluation. The physical therapist recognized that Alex's needs would not be adequately addressed in the eight visits our health insurance company would cover and suggested that we call the Early Intervention System (EIS), a federal grant-funded program administered at the state level. EIS is an outgrowth of the federal Individuals with Disabilities Education Act, the law that establishes the right to a free and appropriate education for all children with disabilities, and offers procedural safeguards to protect the rights of these children and their parents. Under EIS, services are coordinated and provided, at no cost to the family, for children from birth to age three who are experiencing or at risk of developmental delay.

## Finding—and Giving—Support

Our initial contact with the Early Intervention System was a turning point for us. We could not possibly have survived the following months without the support of the agencies with which our service coordinator involved us. We suddenly had educators, nurses, social workers, and therapists all working together to provide a consolidated treatment plan for all areas of Alex's development. They also provided respite ideas and resources for the well-being of the entire family. The support we received through EIS empowered me to take the first steps toward coping with our changing lives.

It became my mission to channel all the sorrow and anger and fear I was feeling into a productive pursuit. I decided to take responsibility for Alex's care by asking questions, finding information, and discussing the applications to Alex's case with his doctors. I had to be as knowledgeable about Alex's condition as possible, no matter how complex or difficult to digest the material was. I began to search the Internet and medical libraries for hours at a time. I pored over the databases of the National Organization for Rare Disorders, the National Institute of Neurological Disorders, and the National Institutes of Health. I read about every disorder with which Alex's symptoms were associated. I contacted everyone I knew who had any medical expertise. I traveled to internationally acclaimed medical centers to get testing and diagnostic "blitzkriegs."

At the same time, I felt a deep need to connect with others who truly understood my pain and sorrow. I started corresponding with parents all over the world via Internet listservs. I found unparalleled support from these other parents—when I was obsessively spending inordinate amounts of time searching for medical information, a friend who was a veteran "special needs" parent pointed out to me that I needed to think of this as running a marathon, not a 50-yard dash: I needed to pace myself. In turn, I began finding that I was providing as much support to other parents as I was receiving. This parent-to-parent connection has been a tremendously important part of our coping strategy—a network of information, medical and educational resources, and emotional support.

Around that time I also became involved with Project DOCC (Delivery of Chronic Care), an organization that uses family caregivers to give future physicians a real understanding of the impact of chronic illness and/or disability on the family. Developed by three inspirational New York City parents of children with chronic conditions—Maggie Hoffman, Donna Appell, and Nancy Speller—Project DOCC trains families to expand future doctors' perspectives beyond the office and hospital to the home and community, to build collaborative relationships between family caregivers and physicians and other professionals.

My association with Project DOCC has been a source of comfort and healing. Project DOCC has provided me with an opportunity to positively use my experiences, good and bad, to help change the way health care is delivered to children with special needs in my community and beyond. It has been tremendously empowering to become a teacher of future physicians. Over the course of the last five years, I have met other families across the country, all advocating for their children in a variety of public arenas in absolutely amazing ways.

We feel so fortunate to have established these support networks during our search for a diagnosis. Alex was two and a half when doctors at what was then the Scottish Rite Children's Hospital in Atlanta informed us that, based on his symptoms, it was highly likely he had a mitochondrial disorder. [Further information on mitochondrial disorders is available at *www.umdf.org.* ] A deep tissue muscle biopsy could confirm the diagnosis, but it would be months before we would receive the results. We understood this was a genetic disorder, but the specific genetic defect and pattern of inheritance were still unknown; we were clearly at risk of having another child affected by the disease if I were to become pregnant again, they told us.

Waiting for the results of the muscle biopsy was nerve-wracking enough, but our fear and stress were magnified when, several weeks before the report arrived, we discovered that I was pregnant! I was frightened of what might lie ahead, and of our doctors' and family's reactions—but even more I wanted this child, our younger daughter, Meg. It was our support network that carried me through this trying time, and celebrated with Jack and me when our healthy baby girl arrived months later.

Perhaps the most important support I received through Project DOCC and my Internet lists, though, was the example of other parent-caregivers who were smiling and laughing and living. I think that for a period of time, at least initially, I wasn't sure that I would ever want to laugh and live again. I felt an ever-present sense of sorrow and loss—that Alex's life might be cruelly shortened; that he had suffered and would suffer more than many other children; that our time had been filled with seemingly endless tasks related to his medical care and educational planning; that I wasn't able to be the parent I planned to be for my children, the wife I wanted to be for my husband; that life had changed completely and thoroughly in ways I could never have anticipated.

Slowly but deliberately, Jack and I have built a new life. Our time is still very limited, but we have learned to use it wisely. We often have periods of days or even weeks where we feel overwhelmed by the workload, but we are better now at finding and accepting support and deciding which tasks can be held off or even eliminated. We have built strong partnerships with several of Alex's doctors that reap benefits in terms of Alex's quality of life, as well as that of the rest of our family. Most important, I have learned how fragile, temporary, and precious our time with family and friends is. I bear in mind Pearl Buck's advice that "there is an alchemy in sorrow. It can be transmuted into wisdom, which, if it does not bring joy, can yet bring happiness." Alex is happy, and I make a point of finding ways to be happy, too.

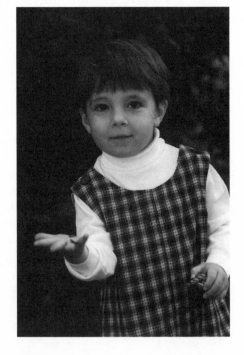

# 8     The Courage of Caring

*Gladys González-Ramos*

So many months have passed and still a dream jolts me from a deep sleep: I enter an old church, the kind that for many years has been a receptacle for people's tears, longings, and prayers. Past the church doors lies a courtyard, with beautiful trees, flowers, and a fountain. It is lush and warm and reminds me of my ancestors' home in Spain. I am looking for my parents among the crowds gathered in the courtyard, but I cannot find them. I stop walking and look down at the outstretched palms of my hands, examining, staring closely at my fingertips as if seeing them for the first time. I begin to feel a pain that becomes so great I can feel it all the way to the tips of my fingers. Then I jolt awake.

In the most exquisite way, my fingertips carry the weight of my loss. Others may not readily see or recognize it, but it remains as alive as ever. When I was a little girl, my mother's soft fleshy arms felt so comfortable that I would often rest against her and fall asleep. She was better than any pillow. My father's tight hugs made me feel secure and loved. What struck me most when I learned that they had died was that I would never feel the tenderness and warmth of their skin. I miss their touch all the way to the ends of my fingers.

In my dream, my hands seem disconnected from my body, just as my loss seems not yet fully integrated into my being. The longing I feel in my outstretched arms continues to this day. Beneath the façade of looking well, my skin continues to feel what I so often miss, and will never have again.

## Neglecting the Patient's and Caregivers' Needs

I write this story as a daughter who cared for her mother, who was diagnosed with Parkinson's disease in 1988, and her father through times of great sorrow and anguish. I also share my story as a social worker and an educator of graduate social work students. Throughout my experience of caregiving for both of my parents, I became acutely aware of how much health care professionals can neglect family caregivers. In light of a devastating chronic illness, it seemed that it became easier for these professionals to narrow their focus to the neurological symptoms of my mother's disease and look past the complex set of emotions she and her family were experiencing. In their myopia they lost sight of her as a whole person.

I do not think that these professionals—physicians, physical therapists, social workers, and others—failed to notice our feelings and multiple needs. They could sense my parents' palpable emotions—loneliness, sadness, fear, anger, and embarrassment, in part at their loss of independence and privacy. At the times when I raised these issues I did not find unsympathetic listeners. Rather, I think that they, too, paralleling our own feelings, felt helpless in light of such enormous complications of body, mind, and spirit. For my mother's symptoms, they felt they could prescribe a medication or some other treatment to alleviate her suffering, and they compartmentalized our feelings and needs as a way of trying to keep them under control.

These professionals underestimated their healing power. They did not seem to understand that listening to caregivers' struggles and feelings can provide much needed relief. They could have helped us tremendously in other simple ways. They could have helped us anticipate what would happen as my mother's illness progressed, what the symptoms would be, and what her day-to-day needs would be. Knowing how to respond would have helped alleviate some of the enormous stress of the unknown. They could have helped by pointing out what services existed, and what options we had at each stage of her illness. These gestures perhaps may seem too simple in light of such enormous need and suffering, but not to inquire, not to delve beyond the neurological symptoms, not to help anticipate the course of my mother slowly losing her abilities—that was worse.

No one knew better than my mother and my father that there was no cure. We did not expect miracles. Rather I, as a daughter, was left to my own resources as a professional social worker to seek out help, services, and advice with the little energy I often had left. We could have received better care—the kind that does not compartmentalize a patient's body and mind while also ignoring the caregivers.

## An Acute Illness, Then a Chronic One

Our story in this country begins when we emigrated from Cuba in 1961. As is the case with most Cuban refugees, we came with no money, as Fidel Castro made sure that anyone who left would not have much to bring with them. We had just the clothes on our backs. I was seven years old and was allowed to bring one doll out of Cuba, but not before the military at the Cuban airport took off the doll's head to make sure my parents were not hiding jewelry or money. My older brother, at age 11, had come to the United States a year earlier because Castro was threatening to remove children from their families and send them away to his own schools. My parents, faced with the many losses of their family, homeland, language, and culture, showed a resiliency and courage that many immigrants find within themselves. They threw themselves into work with fierce determination to make it in this new home. My mother went to work in a factory, and my father did what he knew best—he went into the printing business, working for a Spanish-language newspaper.

Like most immigrants, they struggled and sweated and toiled long, hard hours for the right of freedom and the dream of education for their children. We faced those first few years with fortitude but with poverty as well. We were joined by two other "relatives," whom I referred to as my "aunt" and "grandmother," although they were not blood relations. It was a way to economize and survive life in New York. This arrangement of the six of us living in a small one-bedroom apartment for over two years made my parents even more determined to make it in this country. Through 30 years they prospered in many ways, and eventually opened their own printing business and party goods store.

Within months of their planned retirement my father suffered a sudden, major heart attack, and underwent quadruple bypass surgery. This threw my family and me into a life-and-death emergency, and we pooled our resources to get the best care for my father. After his surgery, he became a model patient. With the same fierce determination he had always shown, he lost excess weight, started to exercise daily, gave up rice and beans, and attended nutrition classes. He would lecture me about nutrition, a role reversal that I found fascinating. He took his perseverance and his work ethic and channeled it into his health, because he wanted to enjoy the rest of his life, travel with my mother as much as they could, and fully enjoy being a grandparent to my brother's three children.

In the midst of his recovery, my mother was diagnosed with Parkinson's disease.

Parkinson's is a neurological disease, one of many movement disorders, which slowly progresses as the brain's nerve cells degenerate, causing the body to lose its capacity for muscular control. This not only affects walking, balance, and large and small muscle movements, but it can also affect bowel movement, urination, and swallowing, among other functions. While most people retain normal intellect, the illness can lead to dementia. About one in every 250 people over age 40 and about one in every 100 people over age 65 will develop Parkinson's. Despite years of research there is no cure. Numerous medications are available, but they all have side effects, which can be quite severe, and as the disease progresses the medications lose their effectiveness (Merck & Co. 1997).

My mother, a strong, healthy woman who had been full of life and known for her kindness and her embrace of a positive spirit, was first diagnosed at age 62. Since she never developed one of the telltale symptoms, a tremor, we later realized that she probably had the illness sometime before the actual diagnosis. At first, the medications the doctors prescribed seemed to greatly improve her ability to move about more easily. Slowly, however, the medications lost some of their effectiveness and my mother's disease began to encroach upon her. As she moved with greater hesitancy for fear of falling, a common occurrence, her world began to shrink. She began to sit and watch television and read more often, and started doing less around the house. She stayed at home more because her muscles might give out on her and she would suddenly have to sit down. Her bladder became affected, so she took increasingly longer in the bathroom because of difficulty urinating. All of these problems made it more complicated to go out and do the simplest of things.

As is typical with the medications available for Parkinson's, side effects increased as the disease progressed. My mother, who had always placed high importance on proper public demeanor, began to suffer from dyskinesias (involuntary bodily movements). The dyskinesias, which could last several hours, caused her to twitch and shake and twist her head. She would experience nausea and eventually vomit, all publicly displayed for people's stares. She would fall off chairs in public, and as we would struggle to pick her up, a mass of "dead weight," I feared the strain would kill my father. She would call herself "un payaso" ("a clown") and try to laugh about it, which only made me want to cry for her, for my father who was so sad, and for myself who felt so helpless.

Until the summer of 1997, when my mother was 71 years old, nine years after the initial diagnosis, my parents managed in their own home. They prized independent living. My mother, who was so attached to her home, did not want any changes to her daily routine. But in September 1997, she deteriorated quite rapidly and began to fall frequently. She became practically wheelchair-bound. We placed her in a nursing home to give her intense rehabilitation following a particularly bad fall and to give my father respite. We also wondered if a good nursing home was a viable alternative at this point.

I, as a social worker and a daughter, had done my homework and thoroughly researched available nursing homes. She went to one that was quite new, modern, clean, bright, and made attempts to be a cheery place. The state reports rated it quite high. But nothing prepared us for the daily experience of a nursing home. It was Halloween time when she was first admitted, so the appropriate ghosts and goblins were displayed in their bright orange and black colors. At first I walked in a daze in the corridors thinking how ironic it was that my parents' party goods store used to sell those very same ornaments. For all the cheeriness that the Halloween goblins tried to provide as they twirled around hanging from the ceiling, what really seeped in was the sadness and loneliness of the patients and their families, even though the staff made every attempt to make it seem like a normal, nice place to live. They had the usual activities of singing, arts and crafts, and even dancing. But the empty, sad stares of the patients too far gone in their minds to know what happy tune might be playing became unbearable.

The nursing home was a nightmare.

Outside of her safe and familiar home environment, my mother sank into depression, surrounded by much older patients with advanced Alzheimer's disease and other dementias. One of the staff psychiatrists evaluated my mother to see if medication could alleviate her depression. The psychiatrist, who did not bother to call my mother's physician or the family, happened to arrive at a time when my mother was having multiple dyskinesias. Seemingly mistaking the symptoms, the doctor prescribed anti-anxiety medication, which only worsened my mother's depression. Once the neurologist took my mother off the anti-anxiety pills, I called the psychiatrist to have her explain why she had prescribed the medication and to see if she had bothered to thoroughly assess my mother's situation or even read her chart before giving her more pills. The psychiatrist, obviously greatly angered by my questioning her judgment, simply said I was not a physician and therefore she could not explain her medical reasoning to me. I realized how little control we had over my mother's care in the nursing home, and wondered about the feasibility of this plan.

My father reacted to placing my mother in a nursing home, and to her growing depression, not by finding respite but rather by spending endless hours by my mother's side trying to take care of her, cheer her up, and provide companionship. In anguish and loneliness, at night he would sob to me on the phone. I would then sob to my husband. My father, who had always been strong, who used to help everyone in the family, whom I had never seen cry, now felt unspeakable loss, and I could find little consolation to offer him.

On a Sunday late in the fall I went to the nursing home and found my father waiting outside the cafeteria for my mother to finish lunch. He was sitting in the bright, modern waiting room quietly crying about my mother's condition. My mother came out of the lunchroom in her wheelchair and started to cry. She was just too sad. She missed her home too much. She missed her life. Then I started to cry because I could not find words to console them. I, too, was beyond words. It was then that we realized this arrangement made no sense. We could not spend the rest of our lives crying in a nursing home. My mother was not better, and my father had gotten no respite. So we took my mother home, with the knowledge that we would hire all the aides that were needed to care for her.

Bringing my mother home meant having to move my parents away from their beloved apartment and the small community in New Jersey where they had lived for more than 20 years. They had a small one-bedroom apartment in a two-story building they owned, which was directly above the business they once owned. This apartment was now unsuitable, as it had a long flight of stairs and was too small to house the several live-in aides we would need. After considering various options, we settled on a two-bedroom, two-bathroom apartment in a building where several family members lived. It was larger, wheelchair-accessible, and closer to my mother's doctors, which was important because transporting her had become increasingly difficult. The other family members nearby could provide ongoing support.

While the move was rationally thought through, it was a great loss, particularly for my father. After my parents retired my father had stayed very active in the community—he had a network of friends, business owners, and associations he belonged to—which gave him a sense of belonging, connection, and purpose beyond his role as a caregiver. Moving from that community touched on his cumulative feelings of being uprooted, harkening back to Cuba. For the first time in their marriage my parents faced a paradoxical situation. What was best for my father—to stay in his apartment, in his community—was not best for my mother.

As I went through my mother's closet to pack her clothes it was like reviewing her life. I found a pocketbook she brought with her from Cuba, the pretty dress she wore to my brother's wedding, all the dresses my father bought her at holiday times, and her pretty, soft, feminine night-gowns. She would never wear these clothes again. Her outerwear had been reduced to easy-to-pull-up pants, which would fit over diapers, and lace-up shoes, which would not fall off during bouts of dyskinesias. There would be little use for a pocketbook since my mother was confined to a wheelchair and could not do much for herself any more.

I wanted my mother to help me, by telling me what I should pack and move, and what I should give away. It was my futile attempt to help her be active and involved. She helped some, until sadness overwhelmed her and she went to another room, leaving the decisions to me. That evening the mourning I felt for my mother struck me particularly deeply. I realized I was losing my mother as I knew her and that I would never have her back again.

That night the lectures I had given to my social work students about "ambiguous loss" became profoundly real to me. I felt conflicted about being in such deep mourning despite the fact that my mother was still alive. I felt guilty for grieving, for I felt I should be thankful that she was still with us. However, the essence of my mother and our relationship was gone. Not only had our roles been reversed, but she was slowly slipping away before my eyes. She was less spontaneous with conversations and could not sustain them for long. All the while she was fully aware of what was happening to her. As Pauline Boss (1999) states in her book, *Ambiguous Loss: Learning to Live with Unresolved Grief*, this is an "unclear loss." She describes how people in my mother's state are "there" yet "not there," physically present but psychologically absent. Such losses, she says, often lead families to experience "frozen grief." Another author describes this experience as an "ongoing funeral" (Kapust 1982). I felt that I was always burying aspects of my mother and our relationship while she was still alive and I was still taking care of her.

During this period I finally convinced my father to seek help. He was drowning in his depression. My parents had always shared a close rela-tionship and had been each other's confidante and best friend. But the progression of my mother's illness made it impossible for her to help my father in decision making, and she could no longer listen to his many sto-ries because of her growing dementia. My father felt he was losing his life partner. He told me that he had slowly accepted her physical limitations but what he missed most about her was her personality. "Se está apagan-do," he would say: "She is fading."

He went to see a psychiatrist, whom I had first talked to and given some brief history. My father needed medication for his depressive signs (lack of sleep and appetite, loss of interest in many things), but more than anything he needed to be listened to. In conjunction with the medication his psychiatrist provided, I wanted my father to see a psychotherapist I had found, who I thought would be good for him, and who could listen to and help him express his sadness and loss. The anti-depressant did relieve some of the outward symptoms, but when the psychiatrist did not return his calls, or would see him for only ten minutes, my father decided not to seek further help. He later promised me he would go with me to see the therapist. We never made it to that visit.

## Bringing on the End

My parents' wedding picture, a simple photograph, conveys the strong bond of love and caring between them. My mother, with a shy smile and in her simple but beautiful dress, at the age of 18 looks youthful but mature beyond her years. She had already endured the deaths of her two parents and two brothers and had spent too much of her youth in hospitals caring for those she loved. My father, 23, so young and handsome in his suit, stands by her side, right behind her, as if guarding her. Nothing about the photograph indicates a wedding: she is not wearing a bridal gown; there are no flowers; there is no cake. They had none of these luxuries when they married. What they had was a great love and a deep commitment to each other, which sustained them through 52 years of marriage.

For my parents' fortieth wedding anniversary we had this photograph refinished and placed in an antique frame, and gave it as a gift at the surprise party we held for them. This picture, as it stood between the two closed caskets at their funeral, reminded us of the strong love and care that brought them together and kept them together at the moment of their chosen death. People at the funeral commented on how right it seemed that their caskets were together, side-by-side, as they themselves had always been in their life.

It was that strong bond and caring that made my father, in a careful, deliberate way, kill my mother and himself, although it is clear that she agreed to it. That fall Sunday afternoon she had been alert and strong enough to understand what he was going to do and did not try to stop him. He had acquired a gun for this purpose, covered her face with a towel, and shot her three times. The medical examiner at the morgue, whom I went to see two months after their death, used words like "caring" and "compassion" to describe the manner in which he killed her, words that don't usually belong to such a violent act.

After shooting her, my father positioned himself by a window of their apartment, sat on the ledge, and shot himself once inside the mouth, the shot propelling his 11-story fall. He landed underneath some bushes, away from nearby parked cars. He chose the particular window well, for if he used any other his body would have landed on someone's car or the parking lot driveway. My father was a man of details, a man who always helped others and never wanted to be a burden. He even carefully orchestrated how to get the two aides out of the apartment during the few precious minutes he needed. He did not want to make it seem that anyone else had been an accomplice.

It is much too easy to judge such actions from a comfortable distance, draw conclusions about motives, and perhaps coat words with professional language. Having read the twenty letters he left behind, the ending seems an act of love, an act of courage, an act of caring.

In his book, *Facing the Extreme: Moral Life in the Concentration Camps*, Tzvetan Todorov (1996) chronicles the lives of people in concentration camps whose caring for one another often led them to choose to die together. He describes a mother, clutching her five-month-old baby who was going to be sent to the gas chamber, who chooses to die with him. He writes about a Dutch woman whose husband was selected to die, who takes his arm and walks with him to their deaths. A man kills his brother, he notes, to prevent his going to the gas chamber. As Todorov states, these people "preferred to take control of their destiny, rather than submit to it passively." In the Warsaw ghetto, he writes, it was "sometimes necessary to kill people precisely because one cared about them."

My father's letters, which he had been writing for several months, provide a window into his thinking and emotions. He tells of the immense sadness he felt, watching my mother slowly deteriorate and suffer through endless bouts of twitching and shaking, with the gradual loss of the ability to swallow. My mother, who had always braved difficulties with fortitude and faith in God, would tell us that she was fine, but her eyes betrayed her unspeakable sadness. The last day I saw her, two days before their death, I had taken her to the doctor. As I hugged her, kissed her, and told her how much I loved her (for there was nothing else I felt I could offer), she looked me straight in the eye and said she loved me and not to worry about her. "I'll be okay," she said. She denied that she felt sad when I asked her, but after her death one of the aides told me that in the last two months she often said that she wanted to die, that she was tired of suffering. My mother had been one of the strong forces in my family; she was not someone who wanted to burden others with her needs and her grief.

My father had been planning this act for over a year; while recognizing how violent it was, he felt it was the only expedient means accessible to him. He would have chosen a quieter way, a physician-assisted suicide, perhaps, but he would have had to include me in the planning as he relied on me for their access to medical care. Once he knew my mother was not a candidate for the available surgeries that might alleviate some of her symptoms, he felt he needed to help relieve her of her misery. He and I often talked about her probable future—a slow deterioration resulting in the loss of her physical functions, and all the while she would be sufficiently alert to know what was happening to her. He explained to me in our multiple daily talks and in the letters that he left behind that he was afraid the stress would bring on another heart attack, perhaps this time fatal. He worried about how my mother would fare in his absence, for even if they no longer slept in the same room, the evening aide told me that my mother endlessly called out my father's name at night when she was in pain or emotional distress.

The last day I spent with my parents remains seared in my mind, for it captures so many of the struggles we had all endured. The drive back to their apartment after the doctor's visit feels as vivid as if it happened yesterday. It was an uncommonly hot and humid fall day, and at noontime we got stuck in one of those maddening Manhattan traffic jams, which lasted more than an hour. Sitting in the front seat of the car, my mother began a bout of dyskinesia, and her movements became more spastic than usual. Unable to control her muscles she grabbed the car's steering wheel and transmission stick. She slowly slid down the seat and wound up with her head and torso on the seat cushion. Her legs pushed up into the air, crushing against the windshield, while her blouse bunched up at her neck so that her brassiere was exposed to everyone's gawking at the many traffic lights where we stopped. As I tried to get her tight grip off the wheel, the aide sitting in the back tried to pull her up and hold her so she wouldn't slip again—a futile task. I tried to calm down my father, who was sitting in the back, agitated, feeling helpless. I have looked back at this endless car ride many times since my parents' death and realized that if my father needed one more maddening moment in which to feel utterly helpless and hopeless, this car ride probably solidified his conviction to end their suffering. This was exactly 48 hours before he ended their lives.

I left my mother at home that day in her special electric chair, her legs propped up in the air, her face showing inexpressible grief. In contrast, as my father walked me to my car, he had a serene smile on his face, which I thought was odd on such a despairing day. As I was about to drive away, on impulse I stopped to give him some cherry-flavored LifeSavers I had in my pocket, for my mother's cough. It was my last act of love, and my last moment in their life. I so wanted to turn all that misery around and make it better for them. All I could do was give my mother my LifeSavers.

It was during another unbearable car ride two days later that I discovered what had happened to my parents. That fateful Sunday I had gone shopping for my mother, who needed additional supplies for her worsening incontinence. As I drove back home with my friend, I called my husband to tell him we were running late. When my cousin answered our phone I knew something was wrong. My husband got on the line and told me my mother was "no longer with us." He didn't want to tell me further details, afraid I would not be able to calmly negotiate the long drive back home. Shaken and stunned, I got off the phone and told my friend that my mother had died. As I sat and thought about it, I shared with her that somehow I knew my father had killed her and then killed himself. I even knew it was with a gun. My father had never owned a gun, was against guns, and yet knowing his determination in life I knew this would have been his way, for it was quick and sure. There was no reason for my mother to die—she was the picture of health, except for the Parkinson's. My father had ended their suffering as a sign of his courage and love. I too got stuck in maddening traffic that night for two hours, luckily with a dear friend, who helped me begin mourning what had just occurred.

### Siempre en Mi Corazón

At their funeral services I, along with my brother, husband, cousins, and nephew, formed the group of 12 pallbearers. I could not bear having paid strangers carry my parents' bodies to their final destinations. I had carried my mother's body in life, when she could no longer hold herself up. I had carried, as much as I could, my father's sadness. I wanted to carry them in their death.

On their gravestones, we had the words "Siempre en Mi Corazón" ("Always in My Heart") engraved. This was my mother's favorite song. They had danced to it at their fortieth anniversary and we played it at their funeral. It begins to capture the unity, love, and caring they formed early in life that carried them together until their death.

## Acknowledgments

I want to acknowledge that I could not have cared for my parents if it had not been for the tremendous support I received from my dear friends. I want to particularly thank my husband, Ernesto Loperena, who held me through these difficult years, cried with me, helped me to carry my mother numerous times, and has always been there with his understanding and love. Thank you also to Pat Hoy for helping me free up my voice and find the way to write this story.

## References

Boss P. 1999. *Ambiguous loss: Learning to live with unresolved grief.* Cambridge, MA: Harvard University Press.

Kapust L. 1982. Living with dementia: The ongoing funeral. *Social Work in Health Care* 7(4): 79-91.

Merck & Co. 1997. *The Merck manual of medical information.* Whitehouse Station, NJ: Merck & Co.

Todorov T. 1996. *Facing the extreme: Moral life in the concentration camps.* New York: Henry Holt & Co.

# 9 The Loneliness of the Long-Term Caregiver

## Carol Levine

I am standing at a bank of phones, desperately punching in codes and numbers. Each time, the line goes dead. "Why can't I get through to anyone?" I think. "I must be doing something wrong."

I wake up. This time it's only a dream. But the dream originated in a real experience. On the icy morning of January 15, 1990, my husband lay comatose in the emergency room of a community hospital after an automobile accident. Uninjured but dazed, I stood at a bank of hospital phones trying to reach people who could help me transfer him to a major medical center. I was unaware that, by a malevolent coincidence, most of the phones in the region were not working.

The dream recurs, and it has now taken on a new meaning. In the nine years since the accident, and especially in the eight years I have struggled to take care of my husband at home, I have frequently despaired: "Why can't I get through to anyone?" Only in the past few years have I realized that I am not doing anything wrong. It is the health care system that is out of order.

Since I have spent 20 years as a professional in the fields of medical ethics and health policy, it is hardly surprising that I should reach such a conclusion. A recent series of articles in the *New England Journal of Medicine* made clear the increasing fragmentation and inequities in the current market-driven health care economy (Angell 1999). But my personal experience as a family caregiver has given me a different perspective. I see the health care system through everyday encounters with physicians,

This chapter originally appeared, with the same title, in the *New England Journal of Medicine*, May 20, 1999, 340(20): 1587-90. © 1999 Massachusetts Medical Society. All rights reserved. Reprinted with permission.

nurses, social workers, receptionists, vendors, ambulette drivers and dispatchers, administrators, home health aides, representatives of my managed-care company, and a host of other "providers." The attitudes, behavior, and decisions of specific individuals make the system work or fail for me.

There are of course critical links between the behavior of individual persons and the system's structural and financial incentives and rewards. Health policy makers and analysts rarely consider the impact of these incentives on the 25 million unpaid, "informal" caregivers in the United States, who get little from the system in return for the estimated $196 billion a year in labor they provide (Arno, Levine, and Memmott 1999). Family caregivers are largely invisible, as individuals and as a labor force.

When my journey began, no one told me what to expect. There is no process of informed consent for family caregivers. On that unforgettable January day, I knew that I must ask, "Is my husband brain-dead?" And I knew what to do if the answer was yes. "No," said the neurosurgeon at the community hospital, "but he has suffered a severe brain-stem injury. At his age [then 62] it is unlikely that he will survive." The neurosurgeon at the medical center disagreed. "He will walk out of here 100 percent, but it will take some time." "How long?" I asked. "Weeks," he replied, "maybe months."

My husband did survive, a testament to one of American medicine's major successes—saving the lives of trauma patients. But he will never walk, and he is far from 100 percent. While he was in a coma, I read to him, played his favorite music, and showed him family pictures. After four months he gradually emerged from the coma, his thinking chaotic. After many more months of relearning basic words and concepts, he recovered many cognitive functions, and there were occasional flashes of his old intelligence and humor. But he is not the same person in any sense.

Although I worried most about his mental functioning, it is his body that has recovered least. He is totally disabled and requires 24-hour care. He is incontinent of bladder and bowel. He is quadriparetic, with mobility limited to the partial use of his left hand. (His right forearm was amputated as a result of an iatrogenic blood clot that failed to respond to surgery and drug treatment.) Even so, the most difficult aspect of his care is his changed personality and extreme emotional lability. Antipsychotic drugs now generally control his violent outbursts, but there are still unpredictable rages and periods of withdrawal.

As a rehabilitation inpatient he had physical therapy, occupational therapy, speech therapy, cognitive therapy, psychological counseling, nerve blocks, injections of botulinum toxin, hydrotherapy, recreational therapy, and therapeutic touch. He benefited to some degree, but nothing restored true function. He has undergone numerous operations, including placement of a shunt after a blood clot formed in his leg, tendon releases in both legs, removal of a kidney stone, and most recently, removal of a pituitary tumor. He has undergone oral surgery and extensive dental work.

During my nine-year odyssey, I stopped being a wife and became a family caregiver. In the anxious weeks when my husband was in the intensive care unit, I was still a wife. Doctors and nurses informed me of each day's progress or setbacks and treated me with kindness and concern. At some point, however, when he was no longer in immediate danger of dying, and as the specialists and superspecialists drifted out of the picture, I became invisible. Then, when the devastating and permanent extent of his disabilities became clear to clinicians, I became visible again.

At that point, I was important only as the manager and, it was expected, the hands-on provider of my husband's care. In retrospect, I date my rite of passage into the role of family caregiver to the first day of my husband's stay in a rehabilitation facility, a place I now think of as a boot camp for caregivers. A nurse stuck my husband's soiled sweat pants under my nose and said, "Take these away. Laundry is your job." A woman whose husband had been at the same facility later told me the same story—different nurse. The nurse's underlying message, reinforced by many others, was that my life from now on would consist of performing an unrelieved series of nasty chores.

The social worker assigned to my husband's case had one goal: discharge. I was labeled a "selfish wife," since I refused to take him home without home care. "Get real," the social worker said. "Nobody will pay for home care. You have to quit your job and 'spend down' to get on Medicaid." Eventually I got the home care I needed—temporarily. Despite a written agreement to pay for it, the insurance company later cut off the benefit retroactively, without informing me, leaving me with an $8,000 bill from a home care agency. The agency, which had failed to monitor its own billing, sued me. We settled for less.

When I brought my husband home, he had undiagnosed severe sleep apnea (which caused nighttime screaming), undiagnosed hearing loss, and poorly treated major depression. The first few months at home were nightmarish. Since the problems had not been diagnosed correctly, much less treated, I did not know where to turn. Yet a single home visit by a psychiatrist and a specially trained home care nurse, arranged by a sympathetic colleague who treats patients with cancer, gave me enough information, advice, and referrals to begin to master the situation.

In addition to holding a full-time job, I manage all my husband's care and daily activities. Being a care manager requires grit and persistence. It took me ten days of increasingly insistent phone calls to get my managed-care company to replace my husband's dangerously unstable hospital bed. When the new bed finally arrived—without notice, in the evening, when there was no aide available to move him—it turned out to be the cheapest model, unsuitable for a patient in my husband's condition. In these all-too-frequent situations, I feel that I am challenging Goliath with a tiny pebble. More often than not, Goliath just puts me on hold.

Being a care manager also takes money. I now pay for a daytime home care aide and serve as the night nurse myself. My husband's initial hospitalization and rehabilitation were paid for by his employer-based indemnity insurance plan. He is now covered by my employer-based managed-care company, which pays for hospital and doctors' bills and, with a $10 co-payment, for prescription medicines. Home care aides, disposable supplies, and most forms of therapy are not covered, because they are "not medically necessary." My husband recently needed a new customized wheelchair, which cost $3,700; the managed-care company paid $500. Medicare, his secondary payer, has so far rejected all claims. No one advocates on my husband's behalf except me; no one advocates on my behalf, not even me.

I feel abandoned by a health care system that commits resources and rewards to rescuing the injured and ill but then consigns such patients and their families to the black hole of chronic "custodial" care. I accept responsibility for my husband's care. Love and devotion are the most powerful motives, but there are legal and financial obligations as well. My income would be counted toward his eligibility for Medicaid, should we ever come to that.

The broader issue of a family's moral responsibility to provide or pay for care is much more complex (Levine 1999). Why should families be responsible for providing such demanding, intensive care? Should this be a social responsibility? American society places a high value on personal and family responsibility. The thin veneer of consensus that supported some sense of communal responsibility in the past is cracking. This is not a uniquely American problem, however. Even with national health insurance, Australian, Canadian, and British caregivers report similar problems of isolation and unmet financial and other needs (Schofield et al.

1998). Only the Scandinavian countries assume that the community as a whole is primarily responsible for long-term care. Even so, the Swedish Social Services Act specifies some spousal responsibility (Barusch 1995).

Widely held concepts of family responsibility derive from religious teachings, cultural traditions, community expectations, emotional bonds, or gratitude for past acts. Caregivers rarely sort out their mixed feelings. From a policy perspective, there are historical antecedents and financial realities that encourage looking first to families for care. Perhaps the most important justification is that most families, or some members, want this responsibility. Many derive spiritual or psychological rewards from caregiving. Taking care of each other comes with being a family. This is an especially strong value among recent immigrants or tightly knit ethnic communities who distrust the formal system but who often have too few resources to cope on their own.

The problem is not that public policy looks first to families but that it generally looks only to families and fails to support those who accept responsibility. The availability of family caregivers does not absolve policy makers of their own responsibility to make sure that their actions assist rather than destroy families. Family members should not be held to a level of moral or legal responsibility that entails jeopardizing their own health or well-being.

Given the complexity of the health care system, what changes would make a difference for family caregivers? The automatic answer tends to be: Whatever they are, we can't afford them. Or, whatever we can afford is not worth doing. Many family caregivers have serious financial problems. Nevertheless, a single-minded focus on money, based on an unsubstantiated assumption that most caregivers want to be replaced by paid help, diverts attention from other critical needs.

The reaction to the Clinton administration's January proposal for assistance for the elderly and family caregivers is an instructive example of the differing worldviews of health policy analysts and family caregivers. Most professionals focused on the proposed tax credit of $1,000 and found it wanting. The credit would not apply to people who pay no taxes, nor would it make a dent in the heavy costs of full-time paid care. The proposal does not do anything to create a coherent long-term care policy (Graham 1999). All these observations are true. On the other hand, family caregivers and organizations that represent their interests have been largely positive about the proposal. The tax credit is a tangible benefit that will help many middle-class families. Equally important, the proposal puts family caregiving on the national agenda and gives states money and incentives to develop resource centers. These points are also all true (Mintz 1999).

In my professional role, I know that much more is needed, including a restructuring of Medicare to better meet the long-term needs of the elderly and disabled and the creation of a more flexible range of options for home and community-based care (Cassel, Besdine, and Siegel 1999). I also know that change will take a long time and will be determined by the interests of the major players and by political considerations. As a family caregiver, I will take whatever help I can get when I need it, and that is right now.

Clinicians as well as policy makers have responsibilities toward family caregivers. Caregivers say they want better communication with professionals, education and training, emotional support, and advocacy to obtain needed services for their relatives and themselves. They want help in negotiating the impenetrable thicket of financing mechanisms, the frequent denials of services or reimbursements, and the inconsistent interpretations of policies and eligibility. They want respite, too, but through services that they can tailor to their needs. These are modest requests— too modest, perhaps—but unfulfilled nonetheless.

Caregivers in the focus groups convened by the United Hospital Fund's Families and Health Care Project reported a lack of basic information about the patient's diagnosis, prognosis, and treatment plan, the side effects of the patient's medication, the symptoms to watch for at home, and whom to call when problems occur (Levine 1998). Sometimes caregivers reported that they were given conflicting information.

Managed care did not create this problem, but it seems to have exacerbated it. Often, professionals convey information in such a hurried, technical way that anxious caregivers cannot absorb it. Hospital staff members may assume, erroneously, that a home care agency will instruct the caregiver. There are costs to these lapses. Failures in communication can lead to serious problems with the care of patients, including unnecessary hospital readmissions. Some families, however, become experts on the conditions of their relatives and the specifics of their care. Yet professionals frequently ignore this expertise, because it comes from laypersons.

Family caregivers also want to be involved in decision making that affects the patient and themselves. Elsewhere (Levine and Zuckerman 1999), Connie Zuckerman and I have described some of the reasons clinicians have difficulties with family members, especially with respect to decisions about acute care (see Chapter 14, "The Trouble with Families: Toward an Ethic of Accommodation"). In my husband's case, I alone made the only important decision, which was to transfer my husband to a medical center on the day of the accident. After that there were never any clear-cut decisions, no discussions about the goals of care, and certainly no long-term planning. Although I repeatedly asked to attend a team meeting to discuss his prognosis and care, I was never given that opportunity. Nor was there ever any follow-up at home, a common complaint among caregivers.

Caregivers want education and training that recognizes their emotional attachment to the patient. Professionals seldom appreciate how much fear and anxiety complicate the learning of new tasks. Learning how to operate a feeding tube or change a dressing or inject a medication is hard enough for a layperson; caregivers learn how to perform these procedures for the first time on a person they love. Fearful of making a mistake or simply upset by the idea of having to perform unaccustomed and unpleasant tasks, caregivers may resist or fail, or persist at great emotional cost.

Months before my husband was ready to go home, a nurse insisted that I learn how to put on my husband's condom catheter. "I don't need to know this yet," I protested, "and besides, maybe he won't need it later." Ignoring our emotional state at the time, she forced me to do it (badly) until both my husband and I burst into tears. Later, when I complained to her supervisor, I was told, "We just wanted to break through your denial."

Families need emotional support. They frequently bring a patient home to a living space transformed by medical equipment and a family life constrained by illness. Privacy is a luxury. Every day must be planned to the minute. The intricate web of carefully organized care can unravel with one phone call from an aide who is ill, an ambulette service that does not show up, a doctor's office that cannot accommodate a wheelchair, an equipment company that does not have an emergency service. There are generally no extra hands to help out in a crisis and no experienced colleagues to ask for advice. Friends and even family members fade away.

Programs that train and support family caregivers can be based in hospitals, community agencies, schools and colleges, home care agencies, managed-care companies, or other settings. The United Hospital Fund's Family Caregiving Grant Initiative is funding several such projects.

If family caregivers need education, professionals need it just as much. Education for doctors, nurses, and social workers should include understanding the needs of family caregivers. Ideally, all professionals should have the experience of seeing firsthand what is really involved in home care. In-service programs can educate health care professionals about family dynamics as well as build communication and negotiating skills.

Family caregivers must be supported, because the health care system cannot exist without them. And there is another compelling reason: Caregivers are at risk for mental and physical health problems themselves. Exhausted caregivers may become care recipients, leading to a further, often preventable, drain on resources. Does my managed-care company realize, for instance, that during the past year it paid more for my stress-related medical problems than for my husband's medical care?

No single intervention will change the system, but small steps taken together can cover a long distance. As I enter my tenth year as a family caregiver, it is hard to believe I have come this far. Today is a reasonably good day. But what about tomorrow? And next week? Hello? Is anyone listening?

## Postscript, 2004

In the years since this article was written and first published, much—and nothing—has changed. For a current perspective on policy initiatives, see Lynn Friss Feinberg's contribution (Chapter 16) in this volume. My husband has survived numerous medical crises and remains at home in much the same condition described in the article. I am still his caregiver, with all the responsibilities and emotional strain that designation entails.

## References

Angell M. 1999. The American health care system revisited—a new series. *New England Journal of Medicine* 340(1): 48.

Arno PS, C Levine, and MM Memmott. 1999. The economic value of informal caregiving. *Health Affairs (Millwood)* 18(2): 182-8.

Barusch AS. 1995. Programming for family care of elderly dependents: Mandates, incentives, and service rationing. *Social Work* 40(3): 315-22.

Cassel CK, RW Besdine, and LC Siegel. 1999. Restructuring Medicare for the next century: What will beneficiaries really need? *Health Affairs (Millwood)* 18(1): 118-31.

Graham J. 1999. Halfway measures. *Chicago Tribune,* January 17.

Levine C. 1998. *Rough crossings: Family caregivers' odysseys through the health care system.* New York: United Hospital Fund.

———. 1999. Home sweet hospital: The nature and limits of private responsibility for home health care. *Journal of Aging and Health* 11(3): 341-59.

Levine C and C Zuckerman. 1999. The trouble with families: Toward an ethic of accommodation. *Annals of Internal Medicine* 130(2): 148-52.

Mintz S. 1999. Statement by Suzanne Mintz, President, National Family Caregivers Association, Kensington, MD, January 6.

Schofield H, S Booth, H Hermann, B Murphy, J Nankervis, and B Singh. 1998. *Family caregivers: Disability, illness and aging*. St. Leonards, Australia: Allen & Unwin.

# PART II
# *The Impact of Caregiving*

# 10 From Sadness to Pride: Seven Common Emotional Experiences of Caregiving

*Barry J. Jacobs*

Several years ago, I observed two radically different caregivers tending to sick spouses on a sub-acute hospital unit where I was a consulting psychologist. One of them, a hoarse-throated, haggard man in his seventies, was piteously grieving the impending death of his wife after a long bout of cancer. His voice shook with barely suppressed emotion each time he conversed with her nurses. At her bedside, he sobbed nearly continuously. The other caregiver, a stately, tight-lipped, sixtyish woman attending to the progressive deterioration of her husband from congestive heart failure, sat by him with little trace of any feeling across her calm features. She asked nothing of the staff, as if she felt prepared to cope on her own with whatever course her husband's illness took. Glancing through the doorways at them in their spouses' respective rooms, I could only imagine that the husband-caregiver's emotional displays represented the death throes of a great love while the wife-caregiver's relative coolness bespoke a more distant or even troubled marriage.

Once I became involved in the cases, however, I found that my impressions were wholly wrong. The adult children of the first couple told me that their parents had savagely battled for decades. The husband had refused to take care of his wife at all through most of her cancer treatment; his behavior now was as likely an act of contrition for previous neglect as it was genuine despair. The second couple's marriage, I learned, had rested upon quiet, rock-solid devotion to one another for 40 years. The wife's lack of expression during his decline stemmed not from lack of caring but from its opposite—the assurance that they had said and exhibited their love for one another so truly over so long a time that nothing more needed to be added now. The prospect of death had only brought them to a wordless contemplation of the deeply felt connection between them.

As the American health care system has become more outpatient-focused through the impact of the growth of managed care, family care-givers have taken on greater importance for the care of the disabled and chronically ill. But the capacity of caregivers to meet these increased demands for extended periods of time is often in doubt. Years of selflessly lifting, spoon-feeding, toileting, and comforting can cause caregivers to lose heart, burn out, and break down. Once that occurs, their ability to care for their loved ones is undermined. Sheer exhaustion of energy and spirit may also place caregivers at risk for developing health problems of their own.

Most health care professionals in hospitals, clinics, homes, and other treatment settings understand the principle of supporting family members in their efforts to care for patients. But as my initial misperceptions of the spouses on the sub-acute unit have reminded me in the years since, clinicians often misjudge caregivers' emotional states. We sometimes believe they are more confident or committed than they really are—the easier for a professional to hand off care of a disabled patient. At times, hospital teams overwhelm family members with training and equipment to send patients home, but later find their plans have failed because they did not pay attention to the family's willingness or capabilities.

At other times, clinicians mistakenly assume that caregivers are downtrodden or depressed because of their self-sacrifices. For instance, we may glibly push a caregiver to "get out of the house and do something for yourself," when what she feels is that caring for her loved one in their home gives her the utmost spiritual gratification. Clinicians' responses, however well-meaning or grounded in sound theories, can badly miss the mark of a given caregiver's makeup and desires.

As numerous commentators (e.g., Wright, Watson, and Bell 1996; Rolland 1994) in the field of families and health have pointed out, it is the meanings that family members attribute to a loved one's disability that greatly shape their emotional reactions to providing care for that person. Those meanings arise from a host of sources, such as the nexus of relationships that have existed over time between the patient and his family members, the family's tradition of caring (or not caring) for debilitated members, and the cultural and religious values that guide the family's notions of appropriate behaviors.

For example, the stroke sufferer who has been much beloved by a cohesive family that prides itself on taking care of its own may be viewed as a tragic victim. His family members may experience shock and sadness and then rally around him. The stroke sufferer with a long history of alcoholism and abusive behavior toward family members may be seen by them as having finally received his due. They may react resentfully, victimized once by his drinking and now again by the unwanted burden of caring for him.

It is not so much the objective circumstances of a given caregiving situation that cause a caregiver to suffer from psychological distress as how that caregiver appraises her predicament, researchers (e.g., Zarit, Johansson, and Jarrot 1998; Pearlin et al. 1990) have found. A wife of an Alzheimer's patient, for example, may regard it as her spousal and cherished duty to care for her husband; the sleepless nights and loss of intimate companionship somehow seemingly cause her little emotional duress. The wife of another Alzheimer's patient with similar behavioral and cognitive deficits may feel trapped by the many hours of correcting, cajoling, and keeping watch over her husband; she may consequently feel stressed beyond her reserves.

Empathy is what matters most in supporting caregivers. Clinicians in all care settings, but especially primary care physicians, social workers, case managers, and home care nurses, best serve caregivers when they strive to understand caregivers' unique family histories and the part that caregiving plays in their individual life stories. Doing so makes evident the contexts and rationales of caregivers' emotional experiences and provides the best opportunity for responding empathically. When they feel understood, caregivers feel less alone with their difficult work and more trusting of the clinicians, advocates, policymakers, and other family members who try to help them. When helpers truly understand caregivers, they can provide more relevant suggestions and solutions to caregivers' problems.

## The Emotional Vocabulary of Caregiving

Empathizing with caregivers requires grasping the affective vocabulary of caregiving—the range of normally expectable emotional reactions. Not surprisingly, researchers of caregivers' emotions have largely limited their explorations to those psychological states that may incapacitate a caregiver, making institutionalization of the patient more likely. Researchers have consistently found that caregivers suffer higher rates of depression and anxiety than non-caregiving adults of the same age (Aneshensel et al. 1995; Cavanaugh 1998; Cochrane, Goering, and Rogers 1997; Gallagher et al. 1989; Pruchno and Potashnik 1989).

As important as these findings are—and as much as they bolster the worthy argument that caregivers in general need more support or risk serious consequences—they fail to capture the emotional experiences of the majority of the people who have decided to devote themselves to others' care. Most do not suffer psychopathology. Rather, their different histories, values, and perspectives lead them to a broad spectrum of experiences. Many respond with different feelings at different times during the course of a loved one's illness, or even during the course of a day. Or they may endure different feelings—some seemingly conflicting—all at the same time. Ambivalence about the roles they play is a common and, for some, perpetual stance. Variability and contradictions abound.

To help health care professionals in all care settings better understand caregivers' experiences and emotional needs, what follows is an outline of some of the emotions caregivers typically encounter. While the descriptions are weighted toward the negative end of the affective scale—for the preponderance of caregivers' reactions is, unfortunately, more negative than positive—the illustrations are intended to be as various as the many meanings that caregivers derive from the vital work they do.

### Sadness

When a family member suffers illness or disability, myriad losses result, from the diminishment of the patient to the alteration of the family. It is disturbing to see a loved one rendered physically helpless, particularly if the injury had a sudden onset. But the advent of cognitive deficits, causing changes in the patient's personality and behavior, is generally far more wrenching for families, note researchers (Hooker et al. 1998). When even so simple a task for the caregiver as sharing the events of one's day and being understood is precluded by a patient's dementia, the loss of companionship is profound.

Decreases in functioning, especially intellectual capacity, will also often force patients who were working to retire, creating economic hardships for the family. When other family members shift to shoulder the bread-winning burden while also assisting the patient more at home with daily activities, they suffer dramatically increased workloads and drastically reduced personal time (see Chapter 12, "The Financial Impact of Caregiving"). Cherished family routines—the neighborhood stroll, the fishing trip—disappear. Illness-phobic family friends vanish, robbing the patient and family of supportive links to the outside world. Perhaps the worst loss is that of the feeling of invulnerability. Once touched by chronic disability, the family is stripped of the belief that all will be right with its members. Nothing feels safe again. Dreams of future happiness are obliterated.

In the face of these many losses, it is natural for caregivers to grieve the passing of their pre-illness lives and feel sad about the difficulties that have befallen them and their loved ones. The ability to accept and express this sadness varies widely, though. Some caregivers find relief in tears and take solace from sharing their mournful feelings with others who respond understandingly. Many caregivers, however, feel uncomfortable about experiencing sadness and shame over displaying it. They typically cite several objections:

- *"I don't want to feel sad because it will make me depressed."* There is a common belief that expressing any sadness, a common human response to loss, will somehow place one on the slippery slope toward major depression, a psychiatric disease state that generally entails some degree of incapacitation. To ensure that they are capable of fulfilling their daily tasks, therefore, many caregivers attempt to maintain a "stiff upper lip." I point out to them that occasional crying is not akin to smashing the dike of one's emotional reservoir. Expressing sadness has a salutary effect on most people, relieving tension and making the development of psychopathological depression less, not more, likely. It also usually enables caregivers to approach their duties more flexibly.

- *"I don't want to express sadness because people will think I'm weak."* There is the common apprehension among some caregivers that, if they openly grieve, others will perceive them as self-centered, self-pitying, and insufficiently devoted. I suggest to them that other people are rarely as harshly judgmental as feared and that, if they are, it is usually because they lack comprehension of what caregivers go through. It is often helpful for caregivers to talk with others in similar circumstances, who have also experienced sadness, about the ways illness has changed their families.

- *"What do I have to feel sad about, when I'm not the one who is disabled?"* Some caregivers feel that they are not entitled to feel sadness for themselves because their losses seem minor compared to the physical or cognitive declines of their loved ones. I suggest to them that one individual's suffering never invalidates the losses of another, particularly when the two people are struggling together against the same adversity in order to live as well as possible. Each deserves a modicum of sympathy and sorrow.

- *"I'm afraid that if I express sadness, it will make my loved one feel worse."* There are instances with demented patients when a caregiver's expressions of sadness can have deleterious effects. For example, a 65-year-old woman who was caring for her 87-year-old, Alzheimer's-addled father in her home found that her father reacted to any negative utterance on any topic that she made as if he were responsible for causing her upset; to decrease his agitation, she had to curb her emotional expressions. Oftentimes in families with physically disabled individuals, a caregiver's show of tears will set off a reaction of shame in the care recipient.

  Generally, though, empathizing with the caregiver's sadness is one of the most effective ways that a patient can give back something meaningful to the person who has made sacrifices on his behalf. When a caregiver is willing to take the risk of expressing sadness to a loved one in a non-blaming fashion, it most often results in a greater feeling of communion or shared mission between the two that helps them both feel better understood and supported (McDaniel, Hepworth, and Doherty 1992).

Health care professionals can normalize feelings of sadness and encourage their expression by inquiring about caregivers' emotional experiences, listening empathetically, and offering insights about typical reactions to caregiving. Explicitly stating that sadness is normal and even helpful can grant permission to even stoical caregivers to explore their feelings. Referrals to support groups, where others are sure to have similar feelings, can frequently help caregivers as well. I believe that helping caregivers accept and express their sadness through these means will allow them to better bear the demands made upon them over time and consequently be less likely to burn out.

## Anger

The many losses that make caregivers sad also commonly make them very angry. The sting of being unjustly trapped and beleaguered often lies at the root of this reaction. It is not unusual for caregivers to harbor thoughts that illness should never have been visited upon their family when other families go unscathed; that the burden of care deprives them of basic life pleasures that others take for granted; that their strenuous efforts receive little notice or thanks. There seems to be no recourse for them, so periodically or perpetually they fume.

Caregiver anger also depends in large part upon the relationship between the patient and caregiver that existed prior to the illness. At its simplest, it takes the form of blaming the patient for bringing tragedy upon the family. I remember, for example, the adult son of a long-term smoker who felt furious at her because, after ignoring his pleas to quit tobacco, she developed disabling emphysema that required daily care.

In more complex previous relationships in which the patient took advantage of the caregiver in some way, the prospect of having to care for her long-term tormentor will only compound the caregiver's sense of being exploited and deprived. I recall the 55-year-old wife of a patient with multiple strokes who took him home from the hospital under staff pressure and then promptly abandoned him. I learned later that she had been physically abused by him for years and now simply couldn't stomach caring for him. A 45-year-old woman who had been perennially angry at her husband for quitting jobs and being a poor provider became so incensed when he suffered a disabling heart attack that she divorced him rather than support him financially any longer.

A third type of prior relationship that can breed anger is when the caregiver feels beholden to the patient in some way but resents being imposed upon now. In Edith Wharton's classic novel *Ethan Frome*, a caregiving husband feels compelled to take care of his invalid wife because she had taken care of his mother in the past. Silently seething because he has to wait hand and foot on his shrewish, ungrateful spouse, he seeks the love of another woman as compensation for all he has sacrificed and then attempts suicide when that love is thwarted.

Another source of caregiver anger lies in the present dynamics between the caregiver and patient. A typical caregiver complaint is that "he won't do anything to help me." Sometimes this is literally true: the patient has regressed to a state of greater helplessness than his disability entails and depends like a child upon the caregiver to meet his needs. Sometimes a caregiver has unrealistic expectations about what her loved one is capable of doing. The caregiver, unable to accept and grieve the extent of the patient's deficits, minimizes his limitations and makes impossible demands upon him.

A second complaint frequently heard is that "he doesn't appreciate all I do for him." In many cases, this is undoubtedly so. Demented patients, in particular, sometimes lack the awareness of self and others to experience gratitude. In others, the caregiver may go about her work so stoically as to encourage the patient's dependency and obliviousness to the caregiver's sacrifices.

The greater community of extended family members, friends, neighbors, and professionals is a final, though significant, cause of caregiver ire. Adult children who care for their parents frequently grouse about how little their siblings contribute. Friends who have backed away since the advent of the patient's disability are deemed betrayers. Neighbors are found to be insufficiently interested and supportive. Health care professionals are sometimes judged to understand too little of the patient and family, care too little to want to understand, and offer medical and psychosocial solutions that make too little difference.

Whatever its source, the intensity of a caregiver's anger can range from low-level, internalized grumbling to moderate frustration to full-blown fury. Regardless of its intensity, health care professionals can best help caregivers deal with their anger by taking the following steps:

- *Acknowledge its legitimacy.* Caregivers need to hear that, as with sadness, anger is a normal, expectable response to arduous circumstances. Its appropriate expression can relieve pressure and bolster resolve.

- *Offer advice on expressing anger.* When voiced too vehemently or in a blaming fashion, anger can alienate others who may be of assistance to the caregiver. When directed at the patient, it may cause pain that can exacerbate the loved one's depression, confusion, or agitation. If it is clear that the caregiver is angry about the disease or disability rather than any individual, she may be able to better join with the patient in fighting together against the common foe. She will likely have more success recruiting others in the cause if she does not put them on the defensive.

- *Offer advice on how to handle particular relationships.* In family situations in which there are grievances about disparities in the amount of care different members are providing, family meetings can help individuals verbalize concerns and renegotiate the caregiving plan as fairly as possible. When caregivers chafe at lack of community support, church and civic association leaders may be approached to communicate the family's needs to willing neighbors.

Anger at the patient is best vented in peer venues such as local chapters of the Well Spouse Foundation, a national support group geared for spouses and partners of seriously ill and disabled individuals. It is not uncommon at Well Spouse meetings for participants to rail against the people for whom they provide care—even to wish them dead—with the encouragement of the entire group. The effect is cathartic; caregivers come away feeling unburdened and understood and better prepared to resume their duties.

- *Coach assertiveness.* Anger, when directed in constructive ways, can allow the caregiver to gain some feeling of control over her predicament. Psychotherapists often coach caregivers in raising questions with and asserting their perspectives to other health care professionals in order to ensure that they are responsive to patients' and families' concerns. Other forms of advocacy, such as pressuring insurance companies to cover necessary services or lobbying legislators to increase research funding or advance proposals for long-term care coverage, are also effective means of turning anger to beneficial uses.

## Worry

Once medical calamity has struck, worry among caregiving families is practically endemic. There is the constant fear of change—that the patient's illness will progress or new disabilities strike; that some deficiency in the caregiver's efforts will be blamed for the care recipient's worsening condition; that the caregiver won't be able to sustain herself for long enough, resulting in the loved one's banishment to a nursing home. There is also the dread that the situation won't substantially change—that the loved one will live forever requiring endless care; that the caregiver will be interminably taxed and tried on a daily basis; that there will never be relief from the excruciating caregiving ordeal.

I remember the 72-year-old wife of a man with bilateral leg amputations, heart problems, and other severe complications from diabetes. When her husband's symptoms were relatively quiescent, she worried continuously about what might befall them next, but functioned effectively. When the feared next medical crisis arose—for instance, temporary kidney failure or an infection requiring another amputation—her reactions instantly escalated from manageable worry to the heightened pitch of anxiety. Her days were plagued with franticness, hypervigilance, and irritability. She slept poorly at night because of her agitation, and experienced pains in her chest and arms due to muscle tension. Just when her husband needed her support the most, she was in the worst shape to help him.

Medical availability and reassurance are the best means of alleviating caregiver worry and anxiety. The patient's primary care provider is in the ideal position to supply this assistance. By meeting monthly or bimonthly with the patient and caregiver, the physician or nurse practitioner can allow timely venting of pressing concerns, quell unrealistic fears with authoritative information, prepare the family for likely downturns ahead, and brainstorm ways of reducing caregiving strain. Having their worries acknowledged and addressed regularly in this fashion enables caregivers to react less severely to living with medical uncertainty.

### Guilt

Many writers on families (e.g., Boszormenyi-Nagy and Spark 1984; Hargrave and Anderson 1992) have noted the reciprocal bonds of loyalty that exist among family members. For what our loved ones have done for us, for how much they have cared for us over time, we often feel obliged to care for them at some point in return. It helps explain the extraordinary devotion of most caregivers: having received love from the patient throughout their relationship, they rise to the sad occasion of medical misfortune to give love back.

But such bonds can be enacted by some caregivers in compulsive ways. The sense of obligation to a family member may be so overpowering that any deviation from carrying out care tasks (attending to one's own needs, for instance) becomes a cause for severe self-renunciation. In this tendency lie the seeds of guilt, the most striking of caregivers' emotional reactions.

Other attitudes contribute to this feeling. Many caregivers have strict definitions of the duties that their family roles comprise. The wife of a patient may feel she is supposed to be at his side every moment. An oldest child may feel she is supposed to move her faltering parents into her home. Sometimes, other family members reinforce these attitudes by subtly pressuring primary caregivers to do their all. In many respects, these convictions are laudable. However, they set very narrow parameters with which to judge individual family members' behaviors, allowing little flexibility of choice in what are usually complex and shifting medical and family circumstances. To do anything but devote oneself fully to a loved one's care can risk condemnation from self and family.

In some cases, survivor guilt also comes into play. Particularly with marriages of long duration, a well spouse may practically reproach herself for remaining well if her loved one has fallen ill. She may set constraints on her own life that parallel those that disability has forced upon her husband so the two can still share the same conditions of life. By declining to participate in activities that he has lost the ability to enjoy, she also protects him as much as possible from the humiliating awareness of his disability.

Magical thinking engenders guilt in other ways. A caregiver may hold the notion that there is something that she could have done to prevent the loved one's illness (e.g., force him to go to the doctor more often). Likewise, she may be convinced that her loved one's future medical course may depend to a large degree upon how well she gives care. If she does a bad job, she believes, the patient will fail; if she does a good job, he will thrive. She may even hope to engineer his recovery in defiance of the dour medical opinions they have received. The result of this reasoning, with high stakes hinging upon her performance, is the cementing of the caregiver all the more to caregiving. Relaxing from her duties even momentarily might have an adverse impact upon the patient and expose the caregiver to withering self-blame.

As can be seen with all its permutations, guilt—or efforts to avoid it—frequently dominates caregivers' lives. It causes them to approach their duties with an intensity of purpose and a rigidity of means. Guilt-ridden caregivers are highly resistant to altering routines or accepting help from others, as if doing so constituted dereliction of duty (Jacobs 1997). At the same time, they disparage their own assiduous efforts. Feeling conflicted, they dig in more doggedly, ignoring the wear-and-tear the years of caregiving bring. Neglecting themselves, they imperil their own health and consequently the well-being of the loved ones who depend upon them so completely.

I still wince at the memory of watching a petite, bone-thin, 60-year-old woman with a history of severe cardiac problems gradually pushing a wheelchair in which her enormous husband was splayed like a tranquilized bear. The strain on her face was both physical and emotional. The effort was clearly too much for her, yet she was determined to uphold her duty and refuse help from anyone, even if it meant pushing herself closer toward another heart attack.

It is a daunting challenge to sway that kind of behavior driven by excessive guilt. Confronting caregivers directly about their exaggerated feelings of responsibility or their attendant self-neglect is rarely productive; they generally disregard the advice as lacking a basis in a true understanding of their motivations. The first step in engaging them effectively, then, is to plumb those motivations by eliciting from them the history and values that led them to their guilty stance. What do they feel they owe patients? What does it mean to them to provide care? If caregivers feel that others understand their rationales and are respectful of their choices, then they are less likely to deflect outsiders' perspectives out of hand.

A good second step is to suggest that caregiving is generally a marathon, not a sprint, and that caregivers who learn to pace themselves through utilizing others' aid have a better chance of maintaining their high level of care—and thereby maintaining the patient's health—over the long haul. For caregivers who even partially concur with this, identifying small initial changes they could make to relieve their burden is important.

Other potential steps for decreasing the intensity of guilt include encouraging caregivers to participate in discussion groups about the problems they face and the accommodations they have made for themselves to handle those difficulties, and asking extended family members and even the patient to explicitly express gratitude to a caregiver for providing care while also stating their concerns about the caregiver's well-being.

## Pride

Caregivers' emotional reactions are not only negative. Climbing the steep learning curve of doing transfers, doling out medications, and working feeding tubes can give them enormous confidence in their abilities. Coping with medical crisis after crisis between long stretches of doldrums can generate pride in their perseverance. When a 42-year-old daughter moved her cancer-riddled mother into her home to care for her, she amazed herself with what she could handle. It wasn't just the basic nursing skills she had mastered that gave her pride; it was that she was able to nurture her mother, a generous woman upon whom she had heavily depended. This act of caregiving changed their relationship and also made her feel more like a capable adult than ever before.

But caregiver pride, when lorded over a patient, can be detrimental. Some caregivers find it so gratifying to have command of their families that they tend to encourage regression on the part of patients. A 40-year-old wife of a man who suffered chronic back pain as the result of an industrial accident took such pride in coordinating his medical care, managing the family business, and running the household that she left little opportunity for her husband to play a viable role in the family (Jacobs

1999). He consequently became depressed and more disabled than would be expected from his injury. It was only when she eventually developed her own health problems and had to back off from some of the roles she savored that the patient found himself able to do more around the house and felt better about himself. The moral to be gleaned is that caregiver pride should be tempered with consideration for preserving the patient's highest possible functioning as a valued family member.

## Gratitude

Occasionally, rather than bemoaning their fate caregivers express thanks for it. They revel in the chance to make a crucial difference in others' lives. Some see it as a means to give back to loved ones who have cared for them so well in the past. Others, taking a more explicitly spiritual view, feel privileged to be the instruments of God's love in conveying comfort and hope. The sense of gratitude these caregivers feel appears to make them more resilient in the face of the long years of demanding work.

Take, for example, the 60-year-old woman who had successively taken care of her ailing mother, mother-in-law, father-in-law, and husband, and then decided to bring her demented father into her home to live with her. Instead of reacting bitterly to having had to devote most of her adult years to caring for others, she said that she felt grateful to have been able to do it because caregiving for the people she loved had been the most rewarding experience of her life. It increased her self-worth and imbued her actions with importance. Her health and outlook were never better, nor was her sense of herself more complete, than when she had someone in her care.

## Ambivalence

Clearly, caregiving provokes a wide range of emotional reactions to a complicated life choice involving personal sacrifice to yield family benefit. Most caregivers are likely to experience a mix of emotions about what they do, depending upon whether they are reflecting on their lot at any specific instant as individual beings or as indebted members of their families. One can feel proud and angry simultaneously. One can feel angry about being burdened, then guilty for having felt anger, and then angry again at having been made to feel guilty. The combinations are infinite. A 75-year-old wife of a Parkinson's patient flip-flops constantly between feeling sad about his impaired condition and angry at him for having it.

A son who is wracked with worry about what will happen next to his arthritic father is grateful for the chance to ease his pain.

Caregiver ambivalence is normal but, when intense enough, can create indecisiveness about care decisions. An angry spouse may often think seriously about resorting to placing the patient in a nursing home, but then feel too guilty to ever send in the necessary paperwork. A worried caregiver may pepper a physician with niggling questions, but then resent the doctor's hubris in telling her what to do. Caregivers' behavior can be inconsistent and therefore confusing for other family members and for health care professionals who try to help. Consequently, they may regard the caregiver as more troubled than she is.

Caregivers, though, are not necessarily troubled at all. Their ambivalence, like every other aspect of their emotional experiences, is the culmination of the histories, values, and perspectives they bring to bear on the tasks they do. What appears merely bollixed makes sense when viewed in light of its unique origins and meanings.

Taking the time for attaining this broad view through dialogue about why caregivers do what they do should be undertaken in all health care settings and be the province of all clinicians, but especially primary care physicians, social workers, case managers, and home care nurses. Any institutional program to effectively help caregivers must start from the point of developing the same kind of understanding of the individuals involved. Because caregiving is a supremely emotional act—the giving up of oneself for another—the empathy we extend to each caregiver is the strongest bulwark we can possibly provide for supporting her sacrifices.

## References

Aneshensel CS, LI Pearlin, JT Mullan, SH Zarit, and CJ Whitlatch. 1995. *Profiles in caregiving: The unexpected career.* San Diego: Academic Press.

Boszormenyi-Nagy I and GM Spark. 1984. *Invisible loyalties: Reciprocity in intergenerational family therapy.* New York: Brunner/Mazel.

Cavanaugh JC. 1998. Caregiving to adults: A life event challenge. In Nordhus IH, GR VandenBos, S Berg, and P Fromholt, eds. *Clinical geropsychology.* Washington, DC: American Psychological Association.

Cochrane JJ, PN Goering, and JM Rogers. 1997. The mental health of informal caregivers in Ontario: An epidemiological survey. *American Journal of Public Health* 87(12): 2002-7.

Gallagher D, J Rose, P Rivera, S Lovett, and LW Thompson. 1989. Prevalence of depression in family caregivers. *The Gerontologist* 29(4): 449-56.

Hargrave TD and WT Anderson. 1992. *Finishing well: Aging and reparation in the intergenerational family*. New York: Brunner/Mazel.

Hooker K, DJ Monahan, SR Bowman, LD Frazier, and K Shifren. 1998. Personality counts for a lot: Predictors of mental and physical health of spouse caregivers in two disease groups. *Journal of Gerontology Series B, Psychological Sciences and Social Sciences* 53(2): 73-85.

Jacobs BJ. 1997. At the caregiver support group. *Families, Systems & Health* 15(2): 213-20.

————. 1999. In sickness and health: Good soldier. *Families, Systems & Health* 17(2): 247-52.

McDaniel SH, J Hepworth, and WJ Doherty. 1992. *Medical family therapy: A biopsychosocial approach to families with health problems*. New York: Basic Books.

Pearlin LI, JT Mullan, SJ Semple, and MM Skaff. 1990. Caregiving and the stress process: An overview of concepts and their measures. *The Gerontologist* 30(5): 583-94.

Pruchno RA and SL Potashnik. 1989. Caregiving spouses: Physical and mental health in perspective. *Journal of the American Geriatric Society* 37(8): 697-705.

Rolland JS. 1994. *Families, illness and disability: An integrative treatment model*. New York: Basic Books.

Wright LM, WL Watson, and JM Bell. 1996. *Beliefs: The heart of healing in families and illness*. New York: Basic Books.

Zarit SH, L Johansson, and SE Jarrott. 1998. Family caregiving: Stresses, social programs, and clinical interventions. In Nordhus IH, GR VandenBos, S Berg, and P Fromholt, eds. *Clinical geropsychology*. Washington, DC: American Psychological Association.

# 11 Caregiving and the Workplace

*Gail Gibson Hunt*

*Betty Smith is a 40-something computer programmer for a branch of a large national bank. Besides being a single parent with two teenagers in high school, Betty is caring for her widowed mother, who lives on her own about ten minutes away. Over the past few years, Betty's mom, now aged 79, has suffered from a variety of chronic illnesses—arthritis, diabetes, and asthma—that are gradually worsening. In addition, Betty thinks that her mother is beginning to show signs of memory loss and agitation.*

*Betty has had to take several days off over the past year to accompany her mother to the doctor, as well as to deal with emergencies. On one occasion she was unable to go to a training seminar that would have improved her job skills and might have led to a promotion. Another time she had to cancel a business trip because her mother had a severe asthma attack. Betty also spends considerable time on the phone at the office, checking up on her mother, making appointments for her, and trying to arrange for home care services.*

*Although Betty's supervisor at the bank has been quite supportive so far, she is getting increasingly concerned about Betty's absences, tardiness, and lack of concentration at work—her lack of "presenteeism," as it were. Betty is thinking about asking for a one-month leave of absence, to give her the time to convince her mother to move in with her and to get her mother's house ready for sale. But the bank just announced another merger and there is talk of downsizing.*

*Betty needs her job and likes working. She is a well-trained and valued employee. But she is also a loving daughter, and wants to do the right thing for her mother. She feels trapped by her competing responsibilities and uncertain of what to do and whom to ask for help.*

Workers, especially poor women, have always had to balance work and family responsibilities, as historical accounts of farm and immigrant families in this country eloquently attest (Abel 1995). Nevertheless, quantitative research in this area is relatively recent, and is linked to the increasing number of women in the formal labor force. In the mid-1980s, as stories like Betty's became more common, some employers began to recognize that child care was not the only family issue affecting their employees' ability to be productive on the job. A number of studies, including those by the Travelers Insurance Companies (1985) and Wagner and colleagues (1989), indicated that workers who were also caregivers of elderly relatives were beginning to constitute an important subgroup of employees whose time at work and productivity were being affected by family responsibilities. The Travelers study surveyed the company's own employees, while Wagner's group surveyed 1,370 employees aged 40 and older in three large Connecticut companies.

Although some of these early surveys found that the proportion of employees who were caregivers was as high as 25 percent, subsequent meta-analysis of 17 of these surveys in the late 1980s and early 1990s revealed very low employee response rates and a more probable incidence of 7 percent to 12 percent of the workforce (Gorey, Rice, and Brice 1992). This meta-analysis also noted the variation in definitions of caregiving in the studies.

## The Costs to Employees

Beyond knowing how many workers are also caregivers, it is important to understand the impact of their caregiving on their employment status. Two national telephone surveys by the National Alliance for Caregiving (NAC) and AARP (1997, 2004) are rich sources of information. The 1997 survey was followed by two more in-depth studies of the data, to be discussed later. The 2004 survey of 1,247 caregivers indicated that 59 percent worked full- or part time. Of these working caregivers, 62 percent said that they had had to make some workplace accommodation as a result of caregiving for a person over the age of 50. Accommodations, as the following numbers indicate, ranged from changing a daily schedule to turning down a promotion:

|  | *Percent of Employed Caregivers* |
|---|---|
| Made any one of the changes listed below | 62 |
| Changed daily schedule: went in late, left early, or took time off during work | 57 |
| Took leave of absence | 17 |
| Worked fewer hours, took less demanding job | 10 |

| | |
|---|---|
| Gave up work entirely | 6 |
| Lost job benefits | 5 |
| Turned down a promotion | 4 |
| Chose early retirement | 3 |

In addition, the survey showed a substantial correlation between the level of care being provided and the need for workplace accommodations. Employed caregivers providing the most intensive personal care associated with Activities of Daily Living (ADLs)—bathing, dressing, or feeding, for example—for the most hours per week were more likely to have made work-related adjustments. Thirty-five percent of those who provided the most intensive caregiving for the most hours reported having to give up work entirely, and 41 percent said they took a leave of absence because of their caregiving responsibilities. In addition, certain other conditions—caring for someone with Alzheimer's disease, living in the same household with the person for whom care is provided, helping with two or more ADLs, or being the primary caregiver—increased the likelihood that caregivers had to make workplace adjustments.

In a 1999 follow-up, called the MetLife Juggling Act Study, in-depth interviews were conducted with 55 caregivers from the 1997 NAC/AARP study who had agreed to participate in further research. To participate in this study, caregivers had to have been 45 years or older in 1996, have made some work adjustment due to their caregiving responsibilities, and provide at least eight hours of caregiving, and at least two caregiving tasks, per week (Metropolitan Life 1999). Three-quarters of the caregivers who participated were women; 45 percent were white, 27 percent African American, 26 percent Hispanic, and 2 percent Asian. This was a relatively affluent group with a steady work history. Their reported incomes ranged from under $25,000 annually (29 percent), through $25,000 to $50,000 (38 percent), to $50,000 and above (26 percent), with 7 percent unreported. Three-quarters of the participants had worked for only one employer during their caregiving experience, and nearly two-thirds had worked for 11 years or more for that employer. This level of job stability may indicate inability or unwillingness to change jobs because of caregiving responsibilities.

Of these participants 30 percent reported that caregiving had limited their skills training, while 20 percent reported turning down the opportunity to work on a special project or declining work-related travel. Forty percent felt that caregiving had limited their ability to advance on the job in one or more ways: 29 percent had refused a job promotion, training, or assignment; 25 percent had refused a job relocation or transfer; 22 percent had not been able to acquire new job skills; and 13 percent had not been able to keep up with changes in necessary job skills.

These lost opportunities had a serious financial impact on the caregivers. Nearly two-thirds of the respondents reported that caregiving had cut their earnings. For the 30 respondents who were able to quantify their losses, the average total loss of income was $566,443. In addition, based on respondent data, the Juggling Act study estimated that their Social Security benefits would decrease an average of $2,160 annually, a lifetime loss of $25,494. Among those eligible for pensions and able to provide information about them, estimated benefits would fall by $5,339 annually, or $67,202 over the course of their retirement. Over their lifetime caregivers would lose, on average, $659,139—a substantial sacrifice.

Almost three-quarters of the respondents said that their own health had suffered as a result of caregiving, and nearly half of these respondents reported additional health care costs and increased absenteeism. Despite the high prevalence of health problems, almost half (47 percent) of the employees did not feel that their work had been affected, and 24 percent reported that it had been "somewhat" affected. Sixteen percent said that work had been affected "a lot" and 13 percent said it had been affected "a little."

## Costs to Employers

Although respondents on the whole did not feel that their job performance had been significantly affected by caregiving, employers may see a different picture. Caregiving entails costs to employers from absenteeism, lowered productivity, and workers' failure to advance. To quantify these costs, the MetLife Study of Employer Costs for Working Caregivers (Metropolitan Life 1997) applied findings from secondary analyses of a number of earlier studies' data, which had identified the major effects of caregiving on employee productivity as:

- replacement costs for employees who quit due to caregiving responsibilities;
- costs of absenteeism;
- costs due to partial absenteeism;
- costs due to eldercare crises; and
- extra time spent supervising employees who are caregivers.

Using data on the number of employed caregivers from the 1997 NAC/ AARP caregiver survey and applying the median weekly wage, the MetLife study estimated the aggregate costs of caregiving in lost productivity to U.S. businesses as $11.4 billion per year—a figure that factored in only those caregivers working full time and providing personal, hands-on care. Including long-distance caregivers and those providing support for *Instrumental* Activities of Daily Living, such as taking a relative to doctor appointments, increased the total loss in productivity to *$29* billion per year.

## Types of Workplace Programs

As a result of the early 1980s studies, some national human resource management companies began to include corporate eldercare programs along with the child care programs they were already offering. These companies perceived the potentially significant impact on productivity of such programs, and a new market for their services. A 1998 survey by the Families and Work Institute estimated that 23 percent of businesses with 100 or more employees offer their workers some type of corporate eldercare programs (Families and Work Institute 1998). Among the earliest companies to do so were IBM, AT&T, StrideRite, and Remington Products. The lead taken by Fortune 500 companies continues today; firms with 500 or more employees constitute the highest percentage of those offering eldercare. There are many reasons mid-size and smaller companies lag behind: a belief that corporate eldercare is costly, lack of resources and specialized personnel, uncertainty about how to provide a service, and wariness about getting too involved in employees' private lives.

Because large firms often have employees at multiple sites around the country, many opt to purchase the eldercare benefits they offer from a national vendor that can provide the same service to employees at any site. Typically, this service—termed "enhanced resource and referral"—offers a toll-free number that employees can call to get basic caregiving information or to obtain a quick assessment of their caregiving problems. If the situation warrants it, the employee is then referred to a local resource and referral person working for one of the network of 250 to 300 such agencies around the country under contract to the principal vendor.

This local resource and referral person conducts a more in-depth assessment of the caregiver's and care recipient's needs and then refers them to appropriate local services such as adult day care or respite. It is the caregiver's responsibility to arrange for the services and to pay for them. The local resource person follows up to see if the situation has been resolved and, if not, to suggest other resources. In addition to a network of resource people, national vendors usually offer an array of other elder-care services: supervisory training, caregiving tip sheets, caregiver fairs, workplace support groups, videos on loan, and Web sites. A few vendors skip the step of going through a local resource network and instead use a national automated database of local resources themselves, directly providing this information to caregivers.

More recently, some larger employee assistance programs, which traditionally offer employees counseling for substance abuse and mental health problems, have also begun to offer corporate eldercare services, including limited counseling, hosting of support groups, manager training, and referrals to local aging agencies. A new benefit being offered by some of the more sophisticated large corporations through their enhanced resource and referral programs is care management. For employees with complex and difficult caregiving situations, the company pays for a geriatric care manager to do an in-home assessment, develop a care plan, and then spend one to three hours arranging services. After that, the employee or care recipient can purchase additional hours of care management at a reduced rate.

Besides services purchased from vendors, some corporate eldercare programs include provisions for flextime; job-sharing; leaves of absence; dependent care accounts, which allow employees to pay for dependent care with pre-tax dollars; long-term care insurance; end-of-life programs; and other employee benefits. Most employers offer just a few of these benefits; seldom are eldercare programs comprehensive.

Web sites offering employees (and the general public) resource information, chat rooms, professional advice, and practical tips on caregiving are becoming more common, although caregivers need to be cautious and check out the sites' sources (see Chapters 19, "Connecting Caregivers through Technology," and 20, "On the Quest for Resources"). In the fall of 2002 the Centers for Medicare and Medicaid Services published a workbook for human resource managers of small and mid-size businesses, describing low-cost and no-cost corporate eldercare programs they can institute (Centers for Medicare 2002).

## End-of-Life Programs

To assess corporate responses to the special needs of employees involved with end-of-life caregiving, the Workplace Task Force of the Last Acts Campaign, a national effort sponsored by The Robert Wood Johnson Foundation, conducted a series of studies in 1998 and 1999. The studies included both focus groups and a mail survey of employee benefits directors of medium and large companies, in part to gauge reactions to proposed models for end-of-life programs, as well as interviews with current and past caregivers of persons with terminal illness. Of the 170 companies that responded to the survey, half had 500 to 1,999 employees and half had more than 2,000 employees (Workplace Task Force 1999).

While a small proportion of companies reported that it was "not too important" (12 percent) or "not at all important" (2 percent) to be able to address employees' end-of-life caregiving issues, the majority felt that it was "somewhat" (43 percent) or "very" (41 percent) important. Many companies already had informal or formal policies or programs in place. The most common benefit reported was paid bereavement leave (88 percent); 60 percent had employee assistance programs or paid family or medical leave apart from vacation or personal leave. A third of the companies arranged temporary reassignments during the period of grieving or medical hardship. Only 15 percent offered a legal services program, whether company- or employee-paid. Such programs might deal with advance directives, powers of attorney, Medicaid eligibility, and other legal issues.

Interviewed employees reported that allowing flexible work schedules or the use of accumulated time off for caregiving was typical. The few employees who were not allowed any flexibility reported negative attitudes toward their employers. Conversely, employees who received encouragement and support from colleagues and supervisors felt more positive about their workplace. Nevertheless, caregivers reported a greater need for support—financial, emotional, and practical—than was available. They responded positively to the idea of employer-provided referrals for counseling and information on topics such as hospice or home health care, and educational materials about dealing with end-of-life decisions.

The Workplace Task Force recommended that employers make three types of assistance the highest priority: providing information and educational materials that will help caregivers deal with end-of-life tasks and decisions; accommodating employees' inevitable need to handle caregiving responsibilities during normal work hours; and recognizing employees' emotional needs and supporting them in any way possible. Since day-to-day supervisors are the individuals most likely to know about an employee's caregiving problems, the Workplace Task Force recommended that supervisors be involved in any program development. It also acknowledged that companies will be more likely to adopt low-cost and easy-to-implement activities, such as providing pre-packaged materials and offering training programs. Working with existing partners and services, such as employee assistance programs, local information and referral networks, and national organizations dealing with caregiving issues, will also make companies more receptive, the Task Force noted.

## Family Medical Leave Act

The federal Family Medical Leave Act has been the prime focus of public policy relating to employment and caregiving (see Chapter 16, "Caregiving on the Public Policy Agenda"). Passed in 1993, the Act allows family members to take up to 12 weeks' leave (several states allow more time) to care for new babies or sick children, spouses, or parents, with the assurance that caregivers can return to their jobs afterwards. While this legislation was significant, it has several drawbacks. First and most important, leave is unpaid. This is a major issue for family caregivers who cannot afford to lose income precisely at a time when they are liable to have additional expenses related to caregiving. Second, the Act applies only to companies with 50 or more employees. Finally, although technically leave can be taken in small increments, it is much more cumbersome to arrange a day or a few hours off than it is to take a block of time to care for a new baby.

While there are several ways the Act could be improved, one policy proposal now on the table concerns the use of state unemployment trust funds to pay for leave. Under a new California law, for example, as of July 2004 workers are allowed to take up to six weeks' paid leave each year for care of a new child or seriously ill family member. Funded by employees' contributions to the existing state disability insurance system, the benefit will replace up to 55 percent of wages, up to a maximum of $728 per week. Four other states—Vermont, Maryland, Massachusetts, and Washington—have already proposed legislation to extend unemployment benefits to new parents. Whatever the outcome of those proposals, though, it is moot for family caregivers of ill and disabled people, since paid leave would apply only to new parents.

## Need for Further Research

While most studies have documented the difficulties caregivers experience in maintaining employment, a few have looked at the benefits caregivers derive. Job satisfaction—a sense of accomplishment, interaction with colleagues, intellectual stimulation—can buffer the negative effects of caregiver stress (see Chapter 6, "Family Caregiving: Both Sides Now"). One study found that women employed full time derived more benefit than part-time workers because they spent more time away from caregiving (Martire, Parris Stephens, and Atienza 1997). More studies are needed on the positive effects of employment for caregivers.

Another area that needs further study is the underutilization of existing workplace programs. National vendors typically have utilization rates around 2 percent—many times lower than the lowest estimate of the number of caregivers in the workplace. A study by Wagner and Hunt (1994) compared users and nonusers of corporate eldercare services. The two principal reasons caregivers gave for not using eldercare programs were "I'm coping and don't need to use the program" and "I feel uncomfortable discussing my caregiving issues in the workplace." These responses indicate that many caregivers, as well as employers, have yet to recognize family caregiving as a workplace issue.

Many of the current national vendor programs grew out of the existing child care model and may not meet the vastly different and much more complex needs of employees caring for elderly relatives. Child care programs may be offered on site, while eldercare is provided at home or in a community facility. Child care programs can be organized around children's predictable needs and developmental stages, while elders may have very individualized health care and management needs. Eldercare programs may also not provide an adequate level of services to meet the needs of those employees who are providing the highest level of care and therefore most at risk of quitting or reducing their hours. The culture of a given organization is also a factor: Is it acceptable to bring these issues to the supervisor? Are there suggested ways to work out accommodations with the supervisor that benefit both the employee and the firm and do not unfairly tax the rest of the employees? Does the CEO support balancing work and family? Are there gender inequalities in job expectations?

To date, there have been no real cost/benefit analyses conducted of corporate eldercare programs—that is, evaluations that quantify the productivity of employees before and after they use such programs, or the effectiveness of the programs in helping employees deal with their problems. Such evaluations would help in supporting the business case for corporate eldercare and might encourage smaller businesses to invest in these services as well.

There are also no studies on the impact on work of caregiving for adults under the age of 50. Workers caring for a 35-year-old spouse with multiple sclerosis or for children with head injuries, for example, have never been surveyed on their need for workplace accommodations. Clearly, to design workplace programs that successfully meet the needs of caregivers of a broad range of ill or disabled family members we must have a better understanding of the services that would support them, and ways to encourage them to take advantage of those services.

## References

Abel E. 1995. 'Man, woman, and chore boy': Transformations in the antagonistic demands of work and care in the nineteenth and twentieth centuries. *The Milbank Quarterly* 73(2): 187-211.

Centers for Medicare and Medicaid Services. 2002. When employees become caregivers: A manager's workbook. http://cms.hhs.gov/partnerships/ materials/caregiversbrochure/Final_Workbook_online_version.pdf Accessed July 21, 2004.

Families and Work Institute. 1998. *1998 business work-life study*. New York: Families and Work Institute.

Gorey KM, RW Rice, and GC Brice. 1992. The prevalence of elder care responsibilities among the work force population. *Research on Aging* 14(3): 399-418.

Martire LM, MA Parris Stephens, and AA Atienza. 1997. The interplay of work and caregiving: Relationships between role satisfaction, role involvement, and caregivers' well-being. *Journal of Gerontology* 52B(5): S279-89.

Metropolitan Life Insurance Company. 1997. *The MetLife study of employer costs for working caregivers*. Westport, CT: MetLife Mature Market Group.

———. 1999. *The MetLife Juggling Act Study: Balancing caregiving with work and the costs involved. Findings from a national study by the National Alliance for Caregiving and the National Center on Women and Aging at Brandeis University*. Westport, CT: MetLife Mature Market Group.

National Alliance for Caregiving and the American Association of Retired Persons. 1997. *Family caregiving in the U.S.: Findings from a national survey*. Bethesda, MD, and Washington, DC: National Alliance for Caregiving and AARP.

———. 2004. *Caregiving in the U.S.* Bethesda, MD, and Washington, DC: National Alliance for Caregiving and AARP. www.caregiving.org/04finalreport.pdf. Accessed July 21, 2004.

Travelers Insurance Companies. 1985. *The Travelers Employee Caregiver Survey: A survey on caregiving responsibilities of Travelers employees for older Americans*. Hartford, CT: Travelers Insurance Companies.

Wagner DL, MA Creedon, JM Sasala, and MB Neal. 1989. *Employees and eldercare: Designing effective responses for the workplace*. Bridgeport, CT: University of Bridgeport.

Wagner DL and GG Hunt. 1994. The use of workplace eldercare programs by employed caregivers. *Research on Aging* 16(1): 69-84.

Workplace Task Force of the Last Acts Campaign. 1999. *Research findings from studies with companies and caregivers*. Washington, DC: National Health Council, National Alliance for Caregiving, and the Last Acts Campaign.

# 12 The Financial Impact of Caregiving

*Donna L. Wagner*

Few people plan in advance for their role as family caregiver. For some of the millions of family caregivers in America, caregiving is precipitated by a sudden and often unexpected event, and is inaugurated by an alarming phone call about a fall, stroke, heart attack, or trauma. For many others the signal event is not so dramatic, occurring after a family member's gradual decline into fragility or dementia. Because family caregiving is becoming a "normative" experience for American families, even those who are not caregivers themselves know someone who is managing the care of a parent, spouse, or adult child.

Many of the consequences of family care are apparent. Caregivers are anxious and preoccupied; they have less time and energy for work, leisure, and other family responsibilities; they often suffer from physical and emotional strain. But because many caregivers do not talk about their financial difficulties, both to maintain their privacy and to avoid any suggestion that considerations of money affect their choices when a family member needs help, the economic toll that caregiving can take is often hidden.

Understanding the economic impact of caregiving requires an analysis of both the individual caregiving situation and the social environment in which caregiving takes place. As noted in the Introduction, informal caregivers provide an estimated $257 billion dollars worth of "free" services annually (Arno 2002), an amount equivalent to nearly 20 percent of *total* annual national health care expenditures. Another, and more realistic, assessment of the situation is that family caregivers have made a contribution to society, as well as to their family members, of $257 billion a year—a contribution that they must bear the cost of both now and in the future.

This chapter explores some of the social factors that are involved in family caregivers' contributions to society. Moving from the social to the personal, the chapter then reviews what is known about family financial contributions in the context of caregiving, the opportunity costs associated with caregiving, and the complicated set of exchanges—rife with emotional as well as economic significance—within families.

## The Shift from Formal to Informal Care

In the U.S. and other industrialized nations, health care services for a growing elderly and disabled population have become increasingly "informalized" (Estes and Swan 1992). The responsibility for health care services for the growing number of Americans with chronic, long-term illnesses is shifting from formal—that is, professional or paraprofessional, paid, hospital- or institutional-based—care to home care, largely provided by unpaid family and friends. Our nation's current approach to "managing" the escalating cost of long-term care as the population ages is largely a strategy of shifting the costs from the public balance sheets of government, corporate insurers, and health provider organizations onto the private balance sheets of families.

As Fast and Frederick (1999) suggest, the 80 percent of care provided by family and friends is a cost-saving measure only if the calculation of public cost-savings fails to factor in the costs now borne by the family. In their analysis of caregiver contributions by family and friends in Canada, they estimate that costs shifted from the public sector to the family were between $5.1 and $5.7 billion (1996 Canadian dollars).

Neither the U.S. estimate of $257 billion nor the Canadian estimate includes the actual costs falling on the family through out-of-pocket expenses, opportunity costs, and/or work-related costs. Nor do they include the costs that are being shifted to the employers of working caregivers, in reduced productivity and absenteeism—for the U.S., estimated at between $11.4 billion and $29 billion annually (Metropolitan Life Insurance Company 1997).

Wolf (1999) argues that, in economic terms, family caregiving provides an "efficient" alternative to formal, paid services. Family and other informal caregivers know the care recipient well, are likely to produce a higher quality "unit of service," and are able to provide services that are more precisely tailored to the needs and the preferences of the care recipient. But although the efficiency of family caregiving is compelling in general, this efficiency will be diminished, and in fact eliminated, by increasing dependence on families. Instead, this increased-efficiency argument supports public investment in family caregiving, not continuing the practice of shifting costs from the public to the family. To date such an investment has been marginal at best.

As Chapter 16 in this volume describes, the National Family Caregiver Support Program passed by Congress in 2001 mandates that specific services be available to family caregivers nationwide, but provides limited resources with which to carry out this mandate. Tax credits for family caregivers have been debated and discussed but have not yet been enacted. There are, however, well-received demonstration programs under way around the nation that allow Medicaid recipients, who must be indigent to be eligible, to pay family members or friends to provide personal assistance services, through a cash allowance in lieu of services (Brown and Foster 2000). On a national level, however, there is no coordinated effort to systematically support caregivers or attempt to minimize the costs they incur as a result of their caregiving activities.

## The Limits of Current Insurance Coverage

Many caregivers are dismayed to discover that private insurance and Medicare, the federal program for people over the age of 65, do not cover long-term health care costs. Developed to respond to the costs of acute illness, Medicare does not provide adequate coverage for meeting the needs of people with chronic, debilitating illness (Eichner and Blumenthal 2003). While a significant portion of a patient's hospital and physician bills may be covered, hospitals, driven by reimbursement policies, encourage rapid discharge, either to a sub-acute facility for a short-term inpatient stay or, more likely, to home.

Medicare will cover a stay in a skilled nursing facility after hospitalization if daily nursing and/or rehabilitative services are required; but most older adults prefer to recuperate at home and many resist even a short-term nursing home stay. When a nursing or rehab facility *is* used for short-term care, support and reimbursement for further rehabilitation or maintenance of the gains achieved there are inadequate. Home care coverage under Medicare (and many private insurance policies as well) is limited to those whom strict guidelines define as "homebound" and requiring skilled nursing care (also strictly defined). It is further limited by the shortage of qualified home health care professionals and paraprofessionals. And under Medicare's Prospective Payment System, home care agencies have economic incentives to "close the case" as soon as possible, and may be reluctant to take on patients who will utilize long and costly care (see Chapter 13, "Social Workers, the Health Care Team, and Caregiver Advocacy," for a case study).

On average, Medicare pays for only ten hours of care per week (Medicare Rights Center 2002). Family and friends must provide the remainder of needed care either directly or by paying for additional home care services out of pocket. In a recent survey of family caregivers who contacted the Medicare Rights Center in New York State, 78 percent reported that they were paying out-of-pocket expenses and 63 percent said they were assisting with health-related tasks themselves. As of this writing, the benefits of the 2003 Medicare prescription drug coverage plan are still being debated, and many private insurance plans do not cover medications outside the hospital setting. Some hospitals even limit provision of drugs to those in their formulary, requiring patients who use other drugs, often expensive ones, to provide them on their own.

Providing care for a person with Alzheimer's disease can be particularly expensive because so much of the care is termed "custodial" and is not reimbursed. Families pay out of pocket an estimated 63 percent of the costs of care (Holden 2001). One analysis suggests that the costs of caring for institutionalized and for community-dwelling persons with dementia are the same, when informal care is included in the analysis. In fact for community-dwelling patients, informal caregiving accounts for the majority of costs—an estimated $18,385 per patient, including more than $6,000 worth of caregiving time provided by family members each year and almost $11,000 per year in lost wages (Moore, Zhu, and Clipp 2001). In addition to the value of direct caregiving and lost wages, more than half the caregivers in this study were also paying for formal care services to handle tasks they could not do themselves—on average $86 for ten hours of service a week.

Medicaid, a federal-state program, offers more comprehensive coverage of long-term care services than does Medicare, although coverage varies by state, and the program is heavily weighted toward nursing home care. In order to be eligible for Medicaid coverage, however, many individuals and their spouses must "spend down," since this program is limited to a strictly defined "indigent" population. Many of those who do go through the spend-down process do it reluctantly, and only after other efforts to provide or pay for care have failed. Maximum benefits accrue to recipients who are "dually eligible"—covered by both Medicare and Medicaid. But while many programs serve this needy—but small—population, there are few services available for the much larger category of people above the poverty line but without adequate resources.

With formal support so limited and rigidly defined, family and friends continue to provide a significant amount of necessary care, in some cases including medically complex procedures that previously would have been managed in a hospital setting (Donelan et al. 2002).

Private long-term care insurance is one option to meet the gaps in current coverage. This form of insurance still comprises a small part of the market, but one that is growing. About four million people, mostly the affluent elderly or near-elderly, are now covered by these policies, with some employer- and government-sponsored plans offering this benefit. Although the average age of purchasers is currently 65, it is gradually dropping; since the average age at which purchasers use the insurance is 82, inflation protection is important (Cohen, Weinrobe, and Miller 2002).

As insurers and consumers gain more experience with private benefit packages, the services provided will probably become more responsive to consumer need. Most people who have filed claims so far have been satisfied with their policies, but many still do not feel that their needs are being met (Cohen 2003). Furthermore, there are significant unresolved regulatory issues, as state insurance departments try to control some of the aggressive and misleading practices that characterized the early plans (Lewis, Wilkin, and Merlis 2003). Although long-term care insurance may be appropriate for some individuals, relieving them and their caregivers of some financial burden, it is unlikely to become affordable for the majority of those in caregiving situations (Merlis 2003).

## Negotiating Family Support

Individual caregivers often absorb serious economic losses as a result of their caregiving role. In many cases caregivers continue to make both financial and personal contributions even when alternatives exist. Studies of caregivers have demonstrated that there is not a clear substitution effect between paid/formal and informal services: families do not necessarily stop caregiving when formal services are available. Nor do they always make economically rational decisions about when to provide a service themselves and when to use a paid service.

The care recipient's preference plays a key role in the balance between informal and paid, formal services. As the care recipient and the primary caregiver negotiate the care strategy they will adopt, their emotional ties, joint history, and family expectations and norms are likely to be more important in the final decision making than the objective needs of the care recipient and abilities of the caregiver.

Care arrangements for older family members are particularly prone to these difficult negotiations. Regardless of the older adult's financial capabilities, adult children may be loath to ask a parent to reimburse them for products or services. Families devise elaborate strategies in order to maintain respectful relationships with their older members, and to defer to elders' attitudes and preferences about services. In one case, after her father refused to accept the local aging network's home-delivered meals, an adult daughter arranged for meals to arrive one evening from the local Chinese restaurant, another evening from the pizzeria, and the third from the chicken take-out. The daughter paid for these meals and left instructions for the delivery person to request only a tip, because her father believed that restaurant food was an extravagance. In another case, a son hired a personal care attendant to provide ongoing daily assistance for his mother, and instructed the attendant to inform her that this was a "volunteer" service.

Within these private family negotiations social supports and policies and family realities intersect. Many families find Medicaid's spend-down process intolerable and do what they can to preserve the dignity and financial independence of their older family member. Others, who do not have the ability to make major contributions, watch in dismay as their proud older relatives take the steps necessary to access publicly funded care.

The transfer of funds between generations has a normative direction in our society—from old to young. When this direction is reversed, many families experience discomfort and tension. Older people may find it intrusive to have an adult child offer financial support, resources, or even advice. The offer can be viewed as a metaphor for dependency, and create conflict between elders and their adult children. In other families, however, older adults or chronically ill siblings may expect a transfer of resources although that would impose a burden upon other family members. Regardless of the family culture, exchanges of money or resources can be some of the most difficult transactions families have experienced amongst themselves. Nonetheless, many intergenerational transfers are taking place, each couched within the particular culture of the individual family.

## Out-of-Pocket Spending

Caregivers incur both direct expenses and less obvious, long-term economic consequences. Many caregivers provide out-of-pocket assistance to care recipients themselves, or to pay for needed services or products, or both. Studies suggest that at least half of those providing care to an older person make outlays for items not covered or only partially covered by insurance—including co-payments, prescription drugs, extended rehabilitation services, home or vehicle modification, customized mobility aids such as wheelchairs and lifts, transportation, special foods and nutritional supplements, incontinence supplies and other disposables, and home health aides providing what is deemed "custodial" care. Overall, long-term home care services are the most costly category in terms of price, but prescription drugs now account for 30 percent of all out-of-pocket costs.

The ongoing costs of small replenishable supplies add up as well. In a survey conducted by The Caregivers Advisory Panel, a national consumer group providing feedback and obtaining products from manufacturers, 80 percent of respondents reported that they are the primary purchasers of health-related supplies for older care recipients, with costs ranging from $1,500 annually for incontinence products to $2 per day for nutritional supplements. It is unclear how many of these primary purchasers seek reimbursement from their family members (Wagner and Alper 2002).

In a nationwide survey of caregivers conducted in 2003, the average amount of out-of-pocket spending reported was $200 a month (National Alliance for Caregiving and AARP 2004). Another study (Merlis 2002) reports that families with a member suffering a serious health problem are twice as likely as other families to spend high percentages of their income on out-of-pocket health-related costs. Merlis's analysis suggests that while poor families and those with seriously ill members are most at risk for disproportionately high out-of-pocket costs, nearly one-third of American families spend more than 5 percent of their annual household incomes on health-related expenses, when the costs of their insurance premiums are included.

Long-distance caregivers, those who live more than an hour from the individual they are assisting, are particularly at risk of incurring significant costs. Respondents in one study of long-distance caregivers (Wagner 1997) reported that they had two categories of costs—those associated with visiting and staying in contact with their family members and those related to helping family members meet their needs. The average out-of-pocket costs spent to keep in touch were $196 per month. Nearly one out of five respondents also reported assisting family members to meet their household needs or pay for services, at an average of $202 per month.

Whether local or long distance, many families also make major outlays for long-term care outside the home. Assisted living facilities are usually expensive and, providing little or no skilled care, rarely subsidized by public sources or third-party payers. Some families bear the costs of skilled nursing facilities, to prevent their older relatives from having to relocate to a less expensive institution or become dependent on Medicaid.

In addition to out-of-pocket expenses for health care-related goods and services, many caregivers are providing underlying financial support—either episodic or ongoing—for their family member. In a recent study of working caregivers, nearly half of the respondents reported that they had provided financial assistance, the majority (75 percent) on an ongoing basis, to the older adult they were helping. Women respondents were just as likely to provide financial support as men, and men and women were providing comparable amounts of support, an average of $272 per month (Wagner, Hunt, and DeViney 2003).

The U.S. Census Bureau estimates that 7.2 million people in America provided ongoing financial support for persons outside their households in 1997 (Masumura 2002). The median amount provided was $2,940, or 6.4 percent of total household income. Adults between the ages of 25 and 64 were most likely to be providing support to others; adult children were the largest group of individuals *receiving* support (78 percent), with parents the next largest group of recipients (9 percent). Because the analysis did not include characteristics of recipients it is not clear just how large a portion of the ongoing support was correlated with caregiving.

## Long-term Economic Consequences

Along with suffering immediate financial consequences, caregivers—the majority of whom are working adults—may have to make career choices that work to their long-term financial detriment. Many of those long-term consequences are related to opportunity costs.

Caregiving is an all-encompassing activity and, for many caregivers, a long-term activity as well. Nearly half of all caregivers report that they have been providing care for five or more years. Studies of caregivers report that the intensity of the caregiving situation may vary, but that 20 hours a week is the average. Some caregiving, particularly for a parent, may be episodic and not uniformly intense over time. Other caregiving, for children with disabilities or spouses with serious illness, for example, can continue at a high level of intensity over long periods of time, during which other activities have a low priority.

Many caregivers are required to put their own plans and aspirations on hold. Pursuing an advanced degree or specialized training, taking a higher-paying job or changing careers, working on creative endeavors, having another child, or even getting married may be deferred into the future. A young caregiver for her grandmother, who lives in another state, finds that although she has started her career she has no time for developing friendships, dating, or pursuing her graduate degree. A young man caring for his brother discovers that not only is he having difficulty doing his job, but his long-term intimate relationship is also at risk of disintegration. Even short-term caregivers not faced with intense care situations are forced to establish priorities on their time, their relationships, and their futures.

The impact of caregiving on existing work has been well-documented; it includes reduced productivity, late arrivals and early departures, missed workdays, the need for an unpaid leave of absence, refusal of a relocation or promotion, and leaving the workplace or job market altogether. About 6 percent of all caregivers decide to leave work permanently (National Alliance for Caregiving and AARP 2004). Some of these adjustments have measurable long-term economic effects. Retirement benefits, for example, are based upon lifetime earnings, and workplace accommodations that result in flat or reduced salary levels obviously have both short- and long-term effects that can be estimated. Other decisions related to caregiving—lost promotion opportunities or career advancements caused by reduced productivity, for example—are more difficult to quantify.

Few studies have attempted to estimate the long-term economic effects of caregiving. One recent analysis estimated that as many as 11 percent of women and 6 percent of men were devoting at least 100 hours annually to caregiving and losing an average of 459 hours of work (Johnson and Sasso 2000). Another study, of 55 women caregivers, estimated that work hours lost to caregiving caused an average lifetime loss of wealth of $659,139 (National Alliance for Caregiving and National Center on Women and Aging at Brandeis University 1999).

Bankruptcy can be the final stage of caregiving's financial impact. In 1999 about a half million individuals sought bankruptcy protection, and about 40 percent of them did so because of overwhelming medical bills, their own or a family member's (Jacoby, Sullivan, and Warren 2000). Not surprisingly, those hardest hit were older people and women, especially those who were single parents.

Even without going into bankruptcy, people with heavy medical debt can suffer grave consequences, such as difficulty getting credit, finding housing, getting a job, and achieving other life goals. People who lose their jobs typically lose their health insurance, and an illness in the family can put them in debt at the worst possible time. In one study of the economic effects of serious or terminal illness, 31 percent of families spent all of their savings and 29 percent lost a major source of income (Covinsky et al. 1994). A study of medical debt in three communities (Alexandria, VA, Champaign, IL, and Miami, FL) found that low-income individuals with and without insurance were struggling with comparable levels of medical debt. Multiple, often confusing bills added to the difficulty of understanding what is owed and why. Increasingly, health care providers are adopting more aggressive collection procedures, such as referring bills to collection agencies more quickly and encouraging patients to pay off their bills with credit cards, thus adding to their indebtedness (Access Project 2003).

While most often the patient is the person with the legal responsibility for medical bills, the family is usually the first place to go for assistance. Even if family caregivers are not obligated to pay bills, they may feel a moral obligation to help out their relative financially. And when the caregiver *is* legally responsible, in the case of a spouse, for example, the consequences can be dire. The *Wall Street Journal* chronicled the plight of a 77-year-old retired dry-cleaning worker being dunned by a hospital where his wife had been treated nearly twenty years earlier. When she died in 1993, her husband was faced with paying off a bill that originally amounted to $18,740. Ten years later, with interest and penalties and the hospital attorney's fees, the bill reached nearly $55,000, of which the husband still owed nearly $40,000. Although he managed to pay $16,000 over the years, he was by then seriously ill himself and would never be able to pay off the debt (Lagnado 2003). (After this story appeared, the hospital forgave the debt.)

## Conclusion

Family caregiving can and often does confer exceptional benefits: persons in need of assistance are able to receive ongoing support from those who not only care for them but who also care about them. Society also benefits from family caregiving, as public expenses for health care are diminished by the efforts of unpaid volunteers. These labors of love often involve both immediate and long-term costs for volunteers, however. And in addition to the economic consequences of hands-on assistance, many caregivers also bear out-of-pocket expenses for products and services, and provide ongoing financial assistance as well.

From an economic and societal perspective, family and friends are an efficient source of long-term care, given care recipients' preferences, caregivers' knowledge of care recipients and their needs, and the fact that this care is unpaid. But this ubiquitous source of long-term care, providing an estimated 80 percent of all long-term care services used, is not free. Nor is it likely to be as available in the future.

As we plan for the aging of our society and seek to ensure quality health care services for those who need them, more research on the economics of caregiving is necessary, not only to fully understand the costs for caregivers now, but also to better support families today and in the future.

## References

Access Project. 2003. *The consequences of medical debt: Evidence from three communities.* Boston: Access Project.

Arno PS. 2002. Economic value of informal caregiving. Paper presented at the meeting of the American Association for Geriatric Psychiatry, Orlando, FL.

Brown R and L Foster. 2000. *Cash and counseling: Early experiences in Arkansas. Trends in consumer choice.* Issue Brief No. 1. Washington, DC: Mathematica Policy Research.

Cohen MA. 2003. Private long-term care insurance: A look ahead. *Journal of Aging and Health* 15(1): 74-98.

Cohen MA, M Weinrobe, and J Miller. 2002. *Inflation protection and long-term care insurance: Finding the gold standard of adequacy.* Washington, DC: Public Policy Institute, AARP.

Covinsky KE, L Goldman, EF Cook, R Oye, N Desbiens, D Reding, W Fulkerson, AF Connors, Jr., J Lynn, and RS Phillips. 1994. The impact of serious illness on patients' families: SUPPORT investigators. Study to understand prognoses and preferences for outcomes and risks of treatment. *Journal of the American Medical Association* 272(23): 1839-44.

Donelan K, CA Hill, C Hoffman, K Scoles, PH Feldman, C Levine, and D Gould. 2002. Challenged to care: Informal caregivers in a changing health system. *Health Affairs (Millwood)* 21(4): 222-31.

Eichner J and D Blumenthal, eds. 2003. *Medicare in the 21st century: Building a better chronic care system.* Washington, DC: National Academy of Social Insurance.

Estes CL and JH Swan. 1992. *The long term care crisis: Elders trapped in the no-care zone.* Newbury Park, CA: Sage Publications.

Fast JE and JA Frederick. 1999. Informal caregiving: Is it really cheaper? Paper presented at the International Association of Time Use Researchers Conference, Colchester, England.

Holden K. 2001. Chronic and disabling conditions: The economic cost to individuals and society. *The Public Policy and Aging Report* (National Academy on an Aging Society, Gerontological Society of America) 11(2): 1-4.

Jacoby M, TA Sullivan, and E Warren. 2000. Medical problems and bankruptcy filings. *Norton Bankruptcy Law Adviser* No. 5 (May): 1-12.

Johnson R and A Sasso. 2000. *Parental care at midlife: Balancing work and family responsibilities near retirement*. A report from The Retirement Project of the Urban Institute, Washington DC. www.urban.org/Template.cfm?Section=ByAuthor&NavMenuID=63& template=/TaggedContent/ViewPublication.cfm&PublicationID=6462 Accessed July 21, 2004.

Lagnado L. 2003. Twenty years and still paying. *Wall Street Journal,* March 13: A1.

Lewis S, J Wilkin, and M Merlis. 2003. *Regulation of long-term care insurance: Implementation experience and key issues*. Menlo Park, CA: Henry J. Kaiser Family Foundation.

Masumura WT. 2002. Who's helping out? Financial support networks among American households: 1997. *Current Population Reports* P70-84. Washington, DC: U.S. Census Bureau.

Medicare Rights Center. 2002. *Easing the burden of family caregivers*. New York. www.medicarerights.org/policyframeset.html Accessed July 21, 2004.

Merlis M. 2002. Family out-of-pocket spending for health services: A continuing source of financial insecurity. The Commonwealth Fund. www.cmwf.org/programs/insurance/merlis_oopspending_509.pdf Accessed July 21, 2004.

———. 2003. *Private long-term care insurance: Who should buy it and what should they buy?* Menlo Park, CA: Henry J. Kaiser Family Foundation.

Metropolitan Life Insurance Company. 1997. *The MetLife study of employer costs for working caregivers*. Westport, CT: MetLife Mature Market Institute.

Moore MJ, CW Zhu, and EL Clipp. 2001. Informal costs of dementia care: Estimates from the National Longitudinal Caregiver Study. *Journal of Gerontology* 56B(4): S219-28.

National Alliance for Caregiving and AARP. 2004. *Caregiving in the U.S.* Bethesda, MD, and Washington, DC: National Alliance for Caregiving and AARP. www.caregiving.org/04finalreport.pdf  Accessed July 21, 2004.

National Alliance for Caregiving and National Center on Women and Aging at Brandeis University. 1999. *The MetLife Juggling Act Study: Balancing caregiving with work and the cost involved*. Bethesda, MD: National Alliance for Caregiving. www.caregiving.org/JugglingStudy.pdf  Accessed July 21, 2004.

Wagner DL. 1997. *Caring across the miles: Findings of a survey of long-distance caregivers*. Washington DC: National Council on the Aging.

Wagner DL and P Alper. 2002. The economic impact of family caregiving.

www.thoushalthonor.org/caregiv/econ_impact.html
Accessed July 21, 2004.

Wagner DL, GG Hunt, and S DeViney. 2003. *Gender, work and eldercare: Study find-ings.* Bethesda, MD: National Alliance for Caregiving, prepared for the MetLife Mature Market Institute.

Wolf DA. 1999. The family as provider of long-term care: Efficiency, equity, and externalities. *Journal of Aging and Health* 11(3): 360-82.

# 13 Social Workers, the Health Care Team, and Caregiver Advocacy

*Terry Altilio and Raymond L. Rigoglioso*

In recent years, two perspectives have developed on the role of family caregivers and their relationship to health care providers, with little acknowledgment of their coexistence or of the way they affect the health care system's perception of its responsibilities toward caregivers. One approach, borrowed from the patient empowerment movement, views caregivers as members of the health care team and advocates for patients and themselves (National Health Council 1999). The alternative view of family caregivers originates in the hospice movement, where the family and the patient are together considered the "unit of care" (Medalie et al. 1998).

The concept of the family caregiver as a member of the clinical team has been very influential in the collective thinking of both caregivers and health care professionals. In a health care system that generally fails to meet caregivers' needs, it is not surprising that they have taken action to win greater visibility and some sense of influence. Yet while it may be empowering and essential for caregivers to be involved in all aspects of a family member's care, viewing caregivers as a part of the health care team has a downside: it makes it all too easy for health care professionals to abdicate their ethical responsibility to serve as advocates for patients *and* caregivers.

Clearly, health care professionals need to recognize the crucial role that family caregivers play in patient care. They should respect caregivers' input, engage them in mutual decision making, and learn from their unique perspectives about the patients for whom they care on a daily basis. But health care professionals must remember that caregivers, too, are vulnerable, need ongoing support, and require information and education that allows for informed decision making. Health care providers have a professional obligation to routinely provide this kind of assistance.

Let's put this into further perspective. Health care professionals generally know what to expect in the course of an illness and its anticipated outcome. They know what questions to ask to determine the most beneficial course of treatment. They share a sophisticated understanding of the language that insurance companies use to approve or deny benefits. And, based on their experience and knowledge, they can often predict what caregivers may experience and need when they bring their loved ones home from the hospital—although sharing that information with the caregiver is still far from common.

In contrast, family caregivers are most often lay people, with little medical knowledge. One day they are husbands, wives, partners, or children and the next they find themselves playing the role of nurse, aide, and advocate. Their lives often get turned upside down in providing care for their loved ones. They have poorer mental health outcomes than their peers (Williamson, Shaffer, and Schulz 1998). One study found that caregivers of Alzheimer's patients suffer from depression at two to three times the rate of others in their age group (Haley 1997). Other studies estimate that between 46 and 59 percent of caregivers are clinically depressed, with a larger percentage of female caregivers experiencing and acknowledging depression (Gallagher et al. 1989; Family Caregiver Alliance 2000; Cohen et al. 1990).

Caregivers often experience high levels of stress-related illness, as the demands of caregiving increase and they neglect their own health needs (Wright, Clipp, and George 1993). In fact, they suffer disproportionately from hypertension, cardiac disease, weight gain, and back problems (Kiecolt-Glaser et al. 1991). Elderly caregivers who experience mental and emotional strain related to caregiving are more likely to have higher mortality rates than their non-caregiving counterparts (Schulz and Beach 1999). Caregivers who are physically and emotionally vulnerable are at a profound disadvantage when it comes to advocating for their loved ones and themselves, both in the health care system and with insurance companies. They must count on physicians and nurses for knowledge about the course of their loved ones' illnesses and nursing needs, and on social workers to assess the psychosocial implications of recommended plans of care, in the beginning as they assume the caregiver role and along the continuum of care as changes occur in the emotional and physical well-being of both the patient and the caregiver.

At the same time that caregivers have asserted their desire to be recognized, far-reaching changes have occurred in the health care system. The advent of managed care saw health care institutions and insurance companies playing a significant role in moving a tremendous amount of care out of the hospital and into the home. With a vast cadre of family members and friends now taking on duties—usually willingly but often under pressure—formerly performed by professionals, providers and payers must assume responsibility for assisting these nonprofessional caregivers.

Such efforts do not have to cost tremendous sums of money. Rather, they hinge on the willingness of health care professionals and insurance companies to transcend the familiar, institution-based focus of care and address challenges arising in the home setting, especially when care is being provided over long periods of time. For all professional members of the health care team, this means taking on a greater advocacy role, ensuring that patients and their families obtain benefits to which they are entitled; improving discharge planning; and providing adequate ongoing education and support. For insurers, this means adopting a more flexible approach to benefits, one that acknowledges the health of the caregiver as crucial to the health of the patient. It also means lowering barriers that make it difficult for families and professional caregivers to help patients access their benefits. For the more than 40 million uninsured patients, advocacy involves the long-term goal of changing public policy, while at the same time assisting patients and their caregivers to maximize access to existing free care and resources from health care agencies, religious and community organizations, foundations, and industry.

## Advocating for Fair Insurance Practices

There was a time when patients could generally count on their insurance booklets to explain their benefits. But with the onset of managed care and the introduction of insurance case managers who can authorize or deny coverage based on their own interpretations of policy language, that previous clarity is now hard to come by. Today, health care professionals' advocacy for patients and their family members becomes all the more important in crafting a plan of care.

Health care professionals should encourage the families with whom they work to be as prepared as possible to deal with their insurers. That includes obtaining a copy of the patient's full insurance policy from the employer or insurer, to supplement the limited summary that is often supplied. Without seeing exactly what coverage is stipulated it becomes very difficult to have an informed conversation, challenge an insurance case manager's decision, or negotiate an alternative plan of care.

To ensure that there are no misunderstandings and, if necessary, to have information for an appeal, health care professionals should also encourage patients and families to request all coverage decisions in writing. That may be especially relevant when it comes to questions of home care, since the advent of a Prospective Payment System—payment based on an episode of care for a particular condition, rather than fee for services actually provided—may have created disincentives for home care agencies to accept demanding cases. It is not uncommon for decisions to terminate service to be announced in person, by a visiting nurse, for example, or for denials of service to be issued via phone. In these situations patients and caregivers will need to make a direct request to the insurance representative for a written explanation of the decisions.

Beyond encouraging families to learn exactly what their benefits include, the health care team can be more assertive about ensuring that case managers receive thorough medical, nursing, and psychosocial information that can influence decision making. In recent years some insurance companies have refused to speak with health care professionals directly, speaking instead only with patients or family members, who rarely have the knowledge, experience, or objectivity to present clinical information thoroughly and convincingly. It is important, therefore, to suggest that patients and/or family members request a conference call with the insurance case manager that includes a representative of the health care team.

Patients and family members also need to understand their rights of appeal when a reasonable plan of care continues to be denied. It is critical to be sure the decision maker is a nurse or other clinically trained person, to get that person's name, and to ask to speak with the individual's supervisor or the medical director. A conference call with the most appropriate member of the health care team may, again, be useful. It is also helpful for social workers, in their role as primary advocates and problem solvers, to help families weigh the pros and cons of engaging employers, union representatives, or regulatory agencies to challenge decisions that seem unreasonable.

Even with adequate information and assertive advocacy, there is no guarantee that an insurance company will cover a stated benefit. A policy may ostensibly cover up to 200 home care visits per year, for example, including intermittent skilled nursing visits. But insurance case managers often interpret such benefits as meaning that skilled nursing coverage will be provided until a family member learns the called-for task. This qualification—"until a family member learns the task"—is seldom put in writing. Yet even patients who have purchased catastrophic policies with extensive private-duty nursing coverage have encountered this limitation. With questionable interpretations of policies not uncommon, social workers must be vigilant about encouraging patients and family members to appeal decisions that are inconsistent with a policy's stated coverage or incompatible with a patient's needs.

For the last 19 years, one of us (Terry Altilio) has worked as a hospital-based social worker, and has witnessed tremendous victories for patients and their families when health care providers have been vigorous advocates for appropriate coverage of care. The following cases, drawn from this professional experience, illustrate how a health care team can make the difference between a patient receiving necessary care and being denied it. Of course there are instances when even the most committed advocacy efforts fail, as one of these cases illustrates, but having the health care team's support may be critical to caregivers' feelings that they have done everything possible.

## Case One

*Mr. R. was a 70-year-old businessman who had prostate cancer. His prognosis was good, but he suffered from recurrent infections and intractable pain that resulted in frequent hospitalizations. Upon discharge he was to receive pain medications and intravenous antibiotics, which had to be administered three times a day. Mr. R. could not administer the antibiotics himself, as his hands shook and he could not reach the intravenous port that had been surgically implanted.*

*Although Mr. R. had three insurance policies, including a catastrophic policy that covered extensive private-duty nursing coverage, the insurance case manager and the nursing agency denied a request for a nurse to administer the antibiotics, arguing that Mr. R.'s wife should do it. Mrs. R., a retired teacher, had already foregone many important personal activities to care for her husband, and over time felt increasingly trapped by his illness. She became distraught at the prospect of having to be further tied to him to administer his medication three times a day. Both the R.s valued their independence and argued that it would cause Mrs. R. undue distress and harm to take on such a task.*

*Their health care team did not unanimously support this argument, even though Mr. R.'s insurance provided ample coverage. Biases cut across disciplines. Some physicians and nurses felt it was Mrs. R.'s responsibility as wife to assist her husband. The social worker and nurse practitioner had fewer preconceived conceptions of gender relationships and responsibilities. These differences became less pronounced when the social worker's psychosocial assessment revealed that Mrs. R. had heart problems and seriously feared that the stress of the situation would bring on a heart attack.*

*The team had initially accepted the insurance case manager's decision without considering both the patient's and caregiver's needs. Once the larger picture became clear, however, the newly won support of the entire team lent extra weight to the social worker's negotiations with the insurance case manager, and the coverage to which Mr. R. was entitled was approved.*

It is the shared responsibility of the members of a health care team to be vigilant regarding care for patients with advanced diseases or extensive nursing needs. Our understanding of both the medical and psychosocial aspects of caregiving, and our knowledge and objectivity about each case, mandate that we provide ongoing assessment, support, and care planning for patients and their caregivers. Insurance case managers need to count on the health care team for information, as they do not have the same immediate understanding of the unique aspects of a particular caregiving situation. Their goal of containing costs often results in a denial of coverage for private-duty home nursing, even if a patient's policy includes it. Instead, in situations of life-limiting illness, they advise patients to enroll in hospice programs, which in most instances are reimbursed at a per diem rate.

Case managers do not always understand that the limited resources of hospices and a capitated reimbursement system make it financially impossible for hospices to provide extensive private-duty nursing coverage. Sometimes health care professionals can advocate for a customized plan of care instead, in which patients can access hospice care, with private-duty nursing services or high-tech pain management being paid for through a separate benefit line in their insurance policies. But hospice is not appropriate for all patients with advanced diseases. Many patients and their families do not elect hospice care, for personal, religious, or cultural reasons. Health care professionals should not allow insurance companies to coerce families into accepting hospice enrollment as the only means of receiving needed care. The case of Mr. K. illustrates how such directives can often be inappropriate and insensitive to the wishes of patients and families.

*Case Two*

*Mr. K. was a 63-year-old attorney who had metastatic prostate cancer. Understanding his limited life expectancy, he chose to spend time with his wife, who was considerably younger than he, preparing her for his death. In keeping with the nurturing role he had assumed in their marriage, he taught her to drive and to manage their finances. He created opportunities for them to spend valued time together. He worked as long as he could and, choosing to remain at home, allowed only essential nursing help and equipment into his home to minimize the disruption to his family life.*

*When Mr. K. developed kidney failure, he had an external urinary drainage tube implanted, which required weekly dressing changes and assessment for infection. Although Mr. K.'s insurance included extensive visiting nurse coverage, the case manager approved nursing service only until Mrs. K. learned to change the dressings. The health care team, understanding that such an arrangement was incongruous with the nature of the K.s' relationship, advocated for once-a-week nursing coverage.*

*The insurance company approved the coverage with the caveat that the service be reevaluated each week. Frequent calls by the case manager to Mr. K.'s home, along with the weekly threat of discontinuing this nursing care, caused the couple great suffering and distress. The insurance case manager suggested that Mr. K. enroll in a hospice program. The couple refused because they wished to maintain continuity with their current health care team rather than establish new relationships as death approached. At the couple's request, the health care team advocated to obtain weekly nursing visits for as long as they were necessary. A member of the health care team insisted on speaking with the case manager's supervisor, the insurance plan physician, to resolve the matter once and for all. The request was never granted, but coverage for Mr. K. was approved indefinitely.*

Another area where advocacy has become ever more important is the use of home health aides, who perform such tasks as bathing, cooking, feeding, and assistance with ambulation and range-of-motion exercises. Historically these services, considered extensions of nursing care, have been approved as long as they accompanied an identified skilled nursing need, such as the administration of intravenous pain medications, physical therapy, or management of wounds. In recent years, in an effort to contain costs, insurance companies have restricted authorization of home health aide services even when patients require skilled nursing. Their justification is that supportive home health services don't directly meet skilled nursing needs.

Such arbitrary interpretations of the home health aide benefit, which represent a dramatic departure from standard practice, are questionable and need to be challenged. The following case illustrates the devastating impact on families and patients when insurance companies restrict covered home health care benefits.

*Case Three*

*Mrs. W. was a 32-year-old mother of two who had metastatic lung cancer. In order to receive care at home, which is what she wished, she required a patient-controlled analgesia pump, and the services of a skilled nurse to assess and manage her pain and shortness of breath and to teach energy conservation techniques to enhance her functioning and safety. Her insurance policy read, "Home health care coverage includes part-time home health aide services for up to 12 hours a day," but the insurance case manager refused to authorize such services because they were "custodial," not "skilled." He only authorized limited nursing visits and recommended that the patient enroll in a hospice program if she wanted additional care.*

*For this family, the notion of hospice ran contrary to its religious belief that every aggressive therapy should be tried to prevent or forestall death, and that death should not be discussed with the dying lest they give up hope and die prematurely. Despite extensive efforts by the social worker and clinical nurse specialist to reverse the ruling, the case manager refused to authorize home health aide services. Mrs. W. was discharged to her home and cared for around the clock by her extended family, with only limited nursing visits. The family, who became exhausted, anxiety ridden, and overwhelmed by the end-of-life care she required, eventually brought Mrs. W. back to the hospital, where she died.*

As this case illustrates, even with the advocacy of health care professionals, patients and families still sometimes go without the care and support they need.

For patients with Medicare and Medicaid in particular, home care benefits may be interpreted differently from region to region. Medicaid, as a combined federal and state program, offers benefits that vary widely from state to state. But Medicare too, although a federal program, differs from area to area, with coverage decisions made by regional fiscal intermediaries. Although the Medicare home care benefit requires that a patient be "homebound," that term is interpreted in a number of ways. A person may be "normally unable to leave home," or unable to leave home "without a major effort," and then only infrequently, for short periods of time, to get medical care or for religious services. Brief absences may not affect eligibility, but once again these parameters differ from region to region (Centers for Medicare 2001). The following case illustrates the importance of integrating and interpreting medical information to maximize opportunities for patients and caregivers to receive home care within these parameters.

## Case Four

*Ms. A. was a 66-year-old single woman living alone in a small apartment. She was in the hospital because of an exacerbation of pain due to colon cancer that had metastasized to the liver. Before her hospitalization, a close friend visited her daily, shopped for her, and accompanied her to doctor appointments.*

*Diagnostic studies indicated that Ms. A.'s cancer was spreading, and no further chemotherapy was planned. The hospital discharge plan integrated the skilled nursing services of a visiting nurse, to assess symptoms and medication side effects, plus physical therapy to maximize functioning, and a home health aide to complement and support Ms. A.'s caregiver friend.*

*Ms. A. valued her independence and functioning. Although weak and fatigued she continued to attempt tasks that were important to her. While aware of the seriousness of her illness, she looked forward to having a home health aide who could take her to the park in her wheelchair, and she hoped to feel "comfortable enough to stop in a favorite coffee shop for a cup of coffee."*

*The nurse evaluator from the Medicare-certified home care agency met Ms. A. in her hospital room as she stood by her sink washing her underclothes. The nurse interpreted Ms. A.'s ability to wash clothes and her desire to go to the park and a coffee shop as indications that she was not homebound or seriously enough ill to warrant a home health aide.*

*Ms. A.'s ability to wash a few small items in the sink and her wish to recover some pleasurable and meaningful activities in the face of progressing cancer did not mean she was not "homebound." Leaving her apartment and spending time in the park would, indeed, be a "major effort" that she could not accomplish alone—an effort that, in a holistic sense, might even be interpreted as a healing or spiritual activity.*

*With that broader view of medical care and rehabilitation, the social worker met with the nurse evaluator and her supervisor to reach a shared understanding of Medicare guidelines and palliative care goals, and to reframe Ms. A.'s behaviors and hopes as a function of her personality and drive rather than a signal that she was not seriously ill and in need of home care services. The care was approved and Ms. A. was able to return to her home rather than to an institution, which she did not want and which would have been more costly.*

Without assistance from knowledgeable professionals, laypersons who do not understand the language of medicine, the intricacies of managed care, or the possible alternative care plans that can be arranged can easily fail to obtain the benefits to which they are entitled. In this time of cost cutting, health care professionals who coordinate discharge plans have the obligation to help patients and family caregivers through mediation, negotiation, and advocacy.

## Improving Discharge Planning

Professional standards obligate health care institutions to smooth the transition from hospital to home or another facility by directly assisting patients and family caregivers prior to discharge. As discussed in the discharge planning booklets produced by the National Alliance for Caregiving and United Hospital Fund, the standards of the Joint Commission on Accreditation of Healthcare Organizations (JCAHO) emphasize the need for an informed, timely discharge-planning process that includes information about the patient's medical condition, clinical basis for discharge or transfer, and alternatives.

Whether coordinated by a case manager, nurse, or social worker, a good discharge plan can mean the difference between a family feeling prepared to take on caregiving responsibilities and its being flung into chaos. Many forces currently at work in the health care system have unfortunately undermined adequate discharge planning.

The Patient's Bill of Rights speaks of the right to "participate in all decisions about treatment and discharge from the hospital." Ideally, such decision making implies informed consent and freedom to make choices about care plans (Arras and Dubler 1994). But with shrinking social work departments and fewer discharge-planning staff, hospitals have instead focused on swiftly moving patients out. The result is that truly informed consent is often not realized, and families bring home sicker patients with even less preparation than they once received. At the same time, the vision of patient participation as outlined in the Patient's Bill of Rights overlooks the fact that, after discharge, the patient is not the only consideration. Family members, whose lives are often profoundly altered when a patient comes home, must be included in this process.

A better discharge-planning process, again borrowing from hospice philosophy, views the *family* as the unit of care and accommodates the language, learning needs, and cultural perspective of the unique patient/ family system. Central to this process is the coming together of the family with the health care professionals involved, making sure that one team member is identified as responsible for coordinating, monitoring, and evaluating the discharge plan.

This meeting affirms the significance of anticipated changes in the family system once the patient goes home, and helps the health care team better grasp the complexities of individual circumstances and the need, at times, for alternative discharge-planning options. Such meetings can be used to delineate workloads, analyze caregiving tasks, and determine the ability and availability of family members to meet the patient's needs. Decisions made this way become a responsibility shared by patient, family, and health care team.

When preparing for this meeting, the social worker or other care coordinator must look beyond the patient's covered benefits to a multidimensional assessment and evaluation of whether care at home is psychologically, financially, and physically possible for the family. To help determine this, the following questions are helpful:

- What are the capacities, needs, and current responsibilities of the caregiver and other family members?
- What are the caregiver's emotional, educational, and ongoing support needs?
- How can continuity of care be maximized amid the ongoing changes in health status of a seriously ill or disabled loved one? (Noddings 1994)

In the course of the family meeting, the social worker and medical team should acknowledge and discuss the profound changes and range of emotions that may occur in and between individuals as they make the transition from the role of family member to that of caregiver. Potential physical changes to the home environment should also be discussed: for many, the home that is their refuge and place of comfort and security is transformed by the presence of medical equipment, health care professionals, illness, and disability, resulting in a loss of privacy and intimacy. The ill family member, in fact, returns in a changed condition to a changed environment (Ruddick 1994).

This is the time for an open discussion of the common wisdom that home care is preferable to care in an institution. For many, hospitals and nursing homes conjure up images of "impersonal" surroundings and "intrusive" treatments, while "home" is often associated with security, comfort, freedom, and intimacy (Ruddick 1994). While some families are able to accept and integrate the adaptations and disruptions that home care creates, others find that the loss of privacy, shift in roles, and dependencies that develop are unacceptable and threaten the essential dignity and personhood of the patient or caregiver. In those cases, the "impersonal" care provided in an institution may be preferable, offering relief and the security of ready access to caring medical professionals, and preserving identity and family relationships. Consideration of "best interest" therefore requires that the social worker explore patient and family preferences, pros and cons, and potential alternatives rather than operate on the assumption that care at home is always preferred (Arras and Dubler 1994).

Whether or not home care is elected, but particularly when it is, the health care team has the obligation to provide families with sufficient training and education during the discharge-planning process. This involves more than just a discussion of a patient's medications or a hurried lesson on how to use a complex piece of medical equipment at home. The clinical person responsible for coordinating care must engage patients and families, over time, in a discussion of their financial and emotional resources, training and educational needs, coping skills, cultural considerations, and family dynamics. Sufficient training and education also includes informing families, as realistically as possible, about what they might expect after discharge.

In summary, for successful discharge planning the health care team must:

- Discuss the patient's medical condition and adequately train caregivers to perform caregiving tasks at home;
- Describe to families what they might expect, medically and emotionally, during the course of illness, while acknowledging that it is impossible to predict every potential development;
- Be realistic about whether the patient is likely to recover or for how much additional time the family can anticipate caregiving;

- Emphasize the "normality" of increased anxiety during transitions;
- Discuss what might constitute a crisis warranting medical assistance or additional home care services;
- Offer information about options, community resources, and referrals for meeting practical, financial, and emotional needs of patients and caregivers;
- Acknowledge that the decisions made and discharge plan developed now may need to be reevaluated in a few months;
- Provide families with information on how to reach the appropriate health care professional if they need to change the plan of care or require additional information.

During the family meeting, caregivers have the opportunity and right to veto a plan they consider to be unmanageable, and alternatives can be explored. Families are often relieved to hear that a plan of care set in place at discharge may need to change over time, and that such a change is not the result of anyone's failure or inadequacy.

## Continuity, Education, and Support

Just as illness evolves and changes over time, even the best discharge plan cannot provide for all the emotional, educational, and support needs that family caregivers will have. Caregivers cannot always absorb or master information that is provided in the hospital, as the anxiety surrounding the discharge process often interferes with listening and learning. In some instances, the equipment a caregiver masters in the hospital is different than that provided by home care suppliers. Many times the evolution and outcome of an illness is uncertain, with the result that health care institutions must take a more proactive role in predicting and identifying the needs of patients and families over time, beyond the hospital walls, and in developing mechanisms to respond to those needs.

Education and skills training can come in many forms, including books and pamphlets, hands-on workshops or one-on-one trainings, Internet resources, and community groups. When designing a program to support caregivers, health care institutions should keep in mind that many caregivers who would not attend support groups will participate in educational programs, which meet the need for information and skills training in a less intrusive way (Schmall 1995). The United Hospital Fund's Family Caregiving Grant Initiative, which awarded funds to seven New York hospitals to design and implement programs to assist family caregivers, is the first of its kind and provides a good range of models for health care institutions interested in providing this kind of help (Levine 2003).

In addition to ongoing education, family caregivers need regular contact with health care professionals to help them reevaluate patient needs and to identify ways to ease the isolation and emotional toll that often accompanies long-term caregiving. Studies indicate that caregivers sometimes perceive their loved one's condition differently than the patient does. While a caregiver may feel hopeless or demoralized, the patient, who is actually living the experience, might feel more optimistic. Hopelessness, denial, or depression may well affect the caregiver's ability to objectively assess a patient's condition, reinforcing the need for professional observation, collaboration, and support (Beckham et al. 1995; Madison and Wilkie 1995).

Patients themselves can also experience a tremendous sense of vulnerability, given their dependent state. They may avoid reporting distress to protect their caregivers from greater sadness or anxiety (Clipp and George 1992). As one patient confided, "Whenever my daughter comes into my room, I can see my suffering reflected in her eyes." Patients at home often become highly attuned to their caregivers' emotions, especially anger and fatigue. They sometimes feel the need to hide their symptoms or emotions, or experience unrealistic pressure to get better and resume their prior roles (Ruddick 1994). Caregivers often report that their ill family members direct a tremendous amount of anger toward them, as well, yet will not display such emotion when a professional is present.

Rather than waiting for caregivers to ask for help, which most often happens when they are already in crisis (Family Caregiver Alliance 1990), scheduling predictable, preventive contacts with a health care professional can help both caregivers and patients defuse these kinds of problems. Encouraging respite care, for example, helps both patient and caregiver recreate the natural boundaries that are a part of maintaining relationships. For a caregiver of a dementia patient, a health care professional could help identify activities to ease the loneliness that often results from losing valued collaboration with a spouse or partner. For a caregiver of a patient with sickle-cell anemia, an appropriate intervention might include education for patient and caregiver about the prevention and treatment of pain flare-ups that accompany the disease.

It is not essential or even possible for hospitals to take on the responsibility for meeting all these needs. Support for caregivers can come from numerous sources, ranging from family physicians, who can screen for caregiver stress to prevent burnout and illness, to community, public health, and disease-based groups, such as those listed in Chapter 20. Such organizations offer a variety of services, including referrals, in-person and telephone support groups, hotlines, literature, newsletters, and Web sites. Hospital discharge planners should become familiar with the services available in their communities and identify contact persons at appropriate organizations so caregivers can find a ready source of support beyond the health care team.

## Insurers' Obligations

By virtue of their role in shifting skilled care into the home, health insurance organizations also have obligations to provide ongoing caregiver support. Adopting programs to assist caregivers, it can be argued, is in insurers' own best interests. The cost savings they realize, after all, are largely predicated on a pool of healthy volunteers: when caregivers become ill due to the work of caregiving, or when a lack of support results in preventable patient hospitalizations, these savings may vanish. Yet it will undoubtedly take pressure from health care professionals, advocates, caregivers, and policy makers to bring about needed changes in insurance companies' practices.

One important way insurance companies could ease the pressures on family caregivers and their loved ones would be to remove some of the barriers to accessing covered benefits. They could train their case managers to communicate in clear lay language what benefits policyholders have and do not have. They could also produce written materials using such lay language. By using complex medical jargon, insurance companies set up patients and their families for failure, and advocacy by health care professionals becomes essential for them to access covered benefits.

Insurers could also be more flexible about benefits, reflecting the vast amount of care that is being provided at home. Such an approach might include a menu of options from which patients and families could choose, to best meet their specific care and support needs. Case managers could be vested with the authority to approve home health aide services and weekend respite care to help families manage care at home over the long term. Insurers could begin covering such benefits as placement in day programs, stress management programs, housekeeping services, and transportation to doctor appointments. They could also designate liaisons to family caregivers and patients, professionals who could provide the kind of ongoing assistance, assessments, and referrals to community resources discussed here. Support for research to determine the overall benefits and cost-effectiveness of these approaches, as well as the costs to insurers of sick and overburdened caregivers, is also essential.

As the broader public comes to better understand the vast unmet needs of caregivers, it becomes increasingly difficult for a compassionate society to ignore the challenge to help. For health care facilities and insurance companies, which have moved more and more care out of the hospital, into the home, and onto the shoulders of volunteers, the obligation to help create programs that better support family caregivers is especially clear.

## References

Arras JD and NN Dubler. 1994. Bringing the hospital home: Ethical and social implications of high-tech home care. *Hastings Center Report* 24(5 Suppl): S19-28.

Beckham JC, EJ Burker, JR Rice, and SL Talton. 1995. Patient predictors of caregiver burden, optimism, and pessimism in rheumatoid arthritis. *Behavioral Medicine* 20(4): 171-8.

Centers for Medicare and Medicaid Services. 2001. *Medicare and Home Health Care.* www.medicare.gov/Publications/Pubs/pdf/10969.pdf Accessed July 21,2004.

Clipp EC and LK George. 1992. Patients with cancer and their spouse caregivers: Perceptions of the illness experience. *Cancer* 69(4): 1074-9.

Cohen D, D Luchins, C Eisdorfer, G Paveza, JW Ashford, P Gorelick, R Hirschman, S Freels, P Levy, T Semla, and H Shaw. 1990. Caring for relatives with Alzheimer's disease: The mental health risks to spouses, adult children, and other family caregivers. *Behavior, Health, and Aging* 1(3): 171-82.

Family Caregiver Alliance. 1990. Who's taking care? A profile of California's family caregivers of brain-impaired adults. San Francisco: Family Caregiver Alliance.

———. 2000. California's Caregiver Resource Center System Annual Report, FY 1999-2000. San Francisco: Family Caregiver Alliance.

Gallagher D, J Rose, P Rivera, S Lovett, and LW Thompson. 1989. Prevalence of depression in family caregivers. *The Gerontologist* 29(4): 449-56.

Haley WE. 1997. The family caregiver's role in Alzheimer's disease. *Neurology* 48(5Suppl 6): S25-9.

Kiecolt-Glaser JK, JR Dura, CE Speicher, OJ Trask, and R Glaser. 1991. Spousal caregivers of dementia victims: Longitudinal changes in immunity and health. *Psychosomatic Medicine* 53(4): 345-62.

Levine C. 2003. *Making room for family caregivers: Seven innovative hospital programs.* New York: United Hospital Fund.

Madison JL and DJ Wilkie. 1995. Family members' perceptions of cancer pain: Comparisons with patient sensory report and by patient psychologic status. *Nursing Clinics of North America* 30(4): 625-45.

Medalie JH, SJ Zyzanski, D Langa, and KC Stange. 1998. The family in family practice: Is it a reality? *Journal of Family Practice* 46(5): 390-6.

National Health Council. 1999. *Family caregiving: Agenda for action: Improving services and support for America's family caregivers.* Washington, DC: National Health Council.

Noddings N. 1994. Moral obligation or moral support for high-tech home care? *Hastings Center Report* 24(5 Suppl): S6-10.

Ruddick W. 1994. Transforming homes and hospitals. *Hastings Center Report* 24(5 Suppl): S11-14.

Schmall VL. 1995. Family caregiver education and training: Enhancing self-efficacy. *Journal of Case Management* 4(4): 156-62.

Schulz R and SR Beach. 1999. Caregiving as a risk factor for mortality: The Caregiver Health Effects Study. *Journal of the American Medical Association* 282(23): 2215-19.

Williamson GM, DR Shaffer, and R Schulz. 1998. Activity restriction and prior relationship history as contributors to mental health outcomes among middle-aged and older spousal caregivers. *Health Psychology* 17(2): 152-62.

Wright LK, EC Clipp, and LK George. 1993. Health consequences of caregiver stress. *Medicine, Exercise, Nutrition and Health* 2(4): 181-95.

# 14 The Trouble with Families: Toward an Ethic of Accommodation

*Carol Levine and Connie Zuckerman*

In a series of 42 interviews with hospital counsel and medical staff at hospitals in New York City, respondents were asked what created the most difficult situations in end-of-life care. Nearly everyone immediately declared, "Families." One physician's response was typical: "They're too emotional. They don't understand what's going on" (Zuckerman 1999).

Paradoxically, the same health care system that is uneasy with families could not exist without them. In today's health care economy, family members not only provide emotional support and ordinary assistance, as they did in earlier decades, but they also implement and monitor high-tech procedures at home that just a few years ago were available only from highly trained professionals in hospital intensive care units. Cost containment, the hallmark of managed care, is largely the shifting of cost and care to patients and families.

Conflicts are most likely to occur in an acute care hospital when the patient is seriously ill or dying and the family is in crisis. When families fail to conform to expected behaviors or disagree with medical professionals and among themselves, they are casually labeled *dysfunctional*. Some families truly are dysfunctional in a clinical, not a dismissive, sense. Other families normally function well but cannot cope with the extreme stress of illness and the alien environment of a hospital. They may fail to appear at critical moments or may be unable to make decisions when needed. On the other hand, the dark view that families are impossible to deal with is only one part of the spectrum.

---

This chapter originally appeared, with the same title, in the *Annals of Internal Medicine*, 1999, 130(2): 148-52. Reprinted with permission. Original abstract has been omitted.

Some clinicians and administrators are extraordinarily sensitive to the legitimate needs and interests of families in medical crises, even though institutional and reimbursement policies, lack of time, and regulatory oversight are often barriers to meaningful attempts to engage and support families. Nevertheless, a persistent tendency is evident, in both the literature and the practice of health care delivery, to equate families with trouble.

Some negative presumptions about families derive from Western medicine's almost exclusive focus on the individual patient in codes of ethics, training, and practice. To the extent that modern bioethics has influenced clinical practice, it has reinforced an individualistic approach by stressing patient autonomy. Physicians' primary responsibilities are unequivocally to their patients. Patient autonomy and a physician-patient relationship based on trust and the physician's concern for the patient's welfare are the primary elements in an ethical framework of medical care. Nevertheless, a complete understanding of the patient's personhood must consider the social network that helps define the patient's core identity. Most persons have some deeply meaningful relationships with others who, by traditional definitions or by choice and commitment, count as "family." These are, in Raphael Cohen Almagor's evocative phrase, the patient's "beloved people" (Almagor 1996).

## Roles of the Family as a Source of Tension

One of the most significant sources of tension between medical professionals and families lies in differing perceptions of the roles that family members should play and how they should play them.

### Family Members as Advocates

Fearing that their relative will be neglected or improperly treated and often having had previous negative experiences with the health care system, families may become extremely vigilant when their relative is admitted to a facility. Nearly 60 family caregivers from the New York metropolitan area who attended a series of six focus group meetings reported experiencing severe stress when the patient for whom they cared was admitted to a hospital (Levine 1998). They felt that they had to be present at all times to explain the patient's special needs to staff and to prevent improper or insensitive care. This was particularly true if the patient was elderly or cognitively impaired.

Families who have dealt with chronic illness are likely to monitor medications and procedures rigorously because they are intimately familiar with the patient's care. Yet their expertise is rarely accorded respect. Families are likely to request assistance that they feel is important for the patient but that may be inconvenient for staff or outside the scope of staff members' perceived job definitions.

Families upset institutional routines and authority in ways that patients do not. Hospitalized patients may exhibit "difficult" behavior or attitudes but, by becoming patients, they hand over much of their freedom and a good deal of their identity to the institution. Their options to complain and make changes are usually limited. Families, however, can identify and seek out officials to whom they bring their concerns. They have strength in numbers. Unlike the sick, they are not subject to the vulnerabilities of patienthood; they are, however, extremely vulnerable in other ways, particularly with respect to hospital routines and policies.

Some hospital policies and restrictions are necessary for safety and infection control. Others, however, are designed to maintain a controlled and efficient environment. Families move unknowingly into situations where the rules of protocol and etiquette are strict but unwritten and where enforcement is often unforgiving; they find out that they have blundered only when they are rebuked for having done so.

Some patients are their own best advocates; their families play a subsidiary role. To use Kuczewski's language, these families "assist the patient's thinking," applying the patient's values and life choices to decisions about treatment options (Kuczewski 1996). But for many patients, especially those who are seriously ill or cognitively impaired, the family is their primary point of contact with the health care system. Even for the competent patient, the family is the link to an identity beyond the illness and to a world in which one makes choices about daily living without the constraint of institutional rules.

### Family Members as Care Providers

Family members provide a substantial amount of direct care. As hospitals become short-staffed, family members are increasingly called on to provide considerable direct assistance. One focus group participant reported, with some pride, that nurses had "allowed" her to clean her mother's room and "do everything" for her. Others were more critical of hospital care and complained that they had to clean patients themselves (Levine 1998).

## Family Members as Trusted Companions

Family members play a role as trusted companions, accompanying a relative through the journey of illness and death, bearing witness, and sharing and responding to the patient's experience. Institutional requirements limiting the presence of family members in critical care units or at the performance of such procedures as cardiopulmonary resuscitation become barriers to family participation. Family members see their presence as a sign of their fidelity at a critical moment in the family history. Staff see family members as interlopers and may be concerned that their presence will interfere with procedures or limit their use of "gallows humor," which is commonly used in such tense situations.

## Family Members as Surrogate Decision Makers

The role of family members as surrogate decision makers for incompetent patients has been analyzed extensively. Most commentators, at least in theory, support the idea that family members are likely to know the patient's wishes well and to act in the patient's best interest. According to many, the ideal decision-making process seems to proceed in a rarefied world of the intellect, unencumbered by the complications of culture, religion, personal history, and beliefs, and unpopulated with relatives, friends, or others with whom the patient has shared both good and bad experiences.

These "extraneous" factors are sometimes lumped together under the rubric of "values"; they are given nodding recognition but are implicitly accorded little importance, largely because they are so difficult to define and measure. The reality is that surrogates are often unclear about the real choices available and about how to participate meaningfully in decision making (Dubler 1995). Some studies have shown that family members often do not know the precise wishes of their relatives, although no other group comes closer to correctly judging what the patient would have wanted in a particular situation (Pearlman, Uhlmann, and Jecker 1992; Seckler et al. 1991; Tomlinson et al. 1990; Sulmasy et al. 1998; Zweibel and Cassel 1989).

## Other Sources of Conflict

Underlying some conflicts between caregivers and families is the often unsubstantiated belief that family members who face financial or care burdens will always put their own self-interest above that of the patient. Moreover, clinicians are frustrated when family members disagree about decisions. Similarly, family members are frustrated when members of the medical team disagree or have inconsistent views. Whether the disagreements surface or not, the family is often expected to speak immediately with one voice, without the benefit of a discussion or a full understanding of the implications of the patient's current medical condition.

Few families are perfectly cohesive; overt or hidden tensions are common. Under the stress of a family member's illness, these tensions can erupt. Longstanding but suppressed differences may emerge; new alliances may be forged; forgiveness and closure may be achieved. Although this may be interesting material for psychotherapy or literature, clinicians find it unnerving and distracting. Rather than acknowledging the impact of the illness on the family, many clinicians distance themselves from the sometimes palpable emotional atmosphere. Particularly when a family member is dying, family members seek solace from each other, from their friends and community, and from the medical staff. Yet physicians often see their role as having ended when "there is nothing more to be done." Perhaps to avoid the emotional atmosphere, to assist other patients for whom they feel their expertise can be more beneficial, or simply to write off a "failure," physicians may drift out of the picture. When this happens, family members invariably feel abandoned, and rightly so.

Families represent a challenge to the authority of professionals and institutions; their role as the watchdogs and agents of quality control is especially threatening. As physicians increasingly feel their traditional authority being undermined by managers, ethicists, regulators, courts, and others, they may view the attempts of a family to influence care as particularly egregious. In some cases, the family's viewpoints or decisions are rejected because they seem ill informed or because the patient's best interests are believed to lie elsewhere. In other cases, family challenges may be rejected because the family's relationship with the clinicians has become so adversarial.

A related source of conflict is the professional's fear of litigation from angry family members. They may shield information or prevent family members from observing the direct administration of care lest something go wrong in the family member's presence. In some cases, they may too quickly capitulate to unwarranted family demands. Although there are no guarantees against lawsuits, numerous studies have clearly shown that litigation is less, not more, likely when communication with families and patients is direct and honest (Hickson et al. 1994; Beckman et al. 1994).

Finally, these conflicts are amplified when the family comes from a religious, cultural, or ethnic background that differs from the one that is dominant among providers. If families and professionals *metaphorically* do not speak the same language, consider how much more difficult communication is when they *literally* do not speak the same language. As the United States becomes more diverse and as families with different values and traditions increasingly come into contact with the health care system, both the tensions between and the mutual dependence of families and professionals are likely to increase.

## Recommendations: Toward an Ethic of Accommodation

The responsibilities and burdens of health care continue to be shifted to informal caregivers, creating an urgent need for family-sensitive policies and practices. Working with families means developing an ethic of negotiation and accommodation, a balancing that has been suggested as the basis for the physician-patient relationship (Siegler 1982) and for long-term and home care (Collopy, Dubler, and Zuckerman 1990; Dill 1995). Given the common histories that lead to shared values and reciprocal obligations between patients and members of their family, the development of an ethic that recognizes the varying roles and interests involved and that works toward negotiation and accommodation where interests compete or diverge will provide a strong foundation on which to build solid partnerships among clinicians, patients, and families.

Patients have both interests and preferences. Their interests include the essential aspects of health, well-being, and functioning, such as independence, mobility, and control. Where these basic interests are at stake, the physician's obligation is to respect patient choices. On the other hand, patient preferences include value-laden choices about the way in which these aspects of life are maintained; for example, whether a daughter should give up her job and move an ailing father into her home or whether the father can stay in his own home with paid help. In this context, the well-being and vital interests of family members also come into play. Unfortunately, no simple formula exists that will establish which interests have primacy. Other professionals, such as social workers, family therapists, or clergy, are often helpful in clarifying options and negotiating acceptable arrangements. As a first step, physicians should explore how involved the patient wants the family to be in care and decision making and should explore the expectations of the family with regard to the same subject.

Caregivers in the New York focus groups said that what they need most is understandable, timely information; better preparation and training for the technical and emotional aspects of their role; compassionate recognition of their anxiety, suffering, and hard work; guidance in defining their roles and responsibilities in patient care and decision making; and support for the setting of fair limits on their sacrifices (Levine 1998). We suggest that these needs can be met by practitioners, administrators, instructors, and others through three main avenues: education and skills acquisition, the establishment of partnerships with families, and regular dialogue and communication.

## Education and Skills Acquisition

Building an understanding of family dynamics and illness into educational materials and seminars can enhance both partnership building and ongoing communication. For example, when family members who have had experiences with illness speak at training sessions on AIDS or cancer, the impact can be powerful. It is also useful to elicit feedback from family members after a crisis has passed. In another exercise, clinical staff can be asked to describe their own experiences as family members at a time when a loved one was ill. In many cases, professionals enter the health care field because of an experience with a relative's illness.

Part of the educational process should be to instill a greater appreciation of the changing structure of families and the variety of ways in which people form meaningful commitments. In some cases, this means exploring deep-seated feelings about homosexual partnerships, unmarried couples, mixed-race marriages, and other nontraditional relationships.

Another key aspect of education is learning about the beliefs, traditions, and heritages of the major cultural and ethnic groups in a community. In some cultures, patients expect physicians to communicate directly with families and expect particular family members to be responsible for decision making. At the same time, it is important not to stereotype all families from a particular group. Cultural norms should be discussed but not assumed. Many influences, such as class, length of residence in the United States, degree of acculturation, education, and personal choice may modify cultural identities. Gender stereotypes held by both administrative and clinical staff ( for example, "women are the caregivers" or "men don't cry") can also influence interactions with family members.

Families also need education. Hospitals now have extensive pread-mission materials for patients; these could be supplemented with fam-ily-focused materials, including information on how families can be most helpful to the patient, on the rationale for visiting hours, on how to iden-tify various staff, and on what to expect in terms of the family's direct or indirect participation in the patient's care. Written and audiovisual ma-terials should support, not substitute for, ongoing discussion. Staff can mentally put themselves in the family's place to identify current institu-tional rules that seem meaningless or unnecessarily rigid and can work to change these rules when appropriate.

## Establishing Partnerships

However difficult it may be, it is important to introduce and practice shared responsibility among patients, clinicians, and families. This is es-pecially critical in decisions that involve the direct participation of and burdens on the family. To be successful, such a partnership must, at a minimum, establish certain ground rules. Partnerships are not friend-ships, and the division of responsibility is not always equal. Partnerships should be dynamic and responsive to changing needs and situations (Pletcher and Deal 1993). In planning for hospital discharge, for example, physicians should ensure that family members who take on significant home care responsibilities are given active, ongoing training, consulta-tion, and practical and emotional support.

## Communication

Communication is probably the single most important aspect of work-ing with patients and their families. It involves active listening as well as talking, and it requires both time and patience. Does the family under-stand the severity of the patient's condition? How have they dealt with the diagnosis and prognosis? What are the family's expressed concerns? What questions lie just below the surface? How can mixed messages be avoided? How can information be conveyed consistently and clearly?

Confidentiality and truth telling present particularly thorny challeng-es. Cases in which professional standards of confidentiality conflict with those of patients and families are not easy to resolve, but they can usually be negotiated to an acceptable compromise.

Along with learning communication skills, it is essential that caregivers acquire techniques for minimizing conflict (Butler, Holloway, and Gottlieb 1998). Angry confrontations or sullen indifference on the part of clinical staff often lead to even more aggressive and unpleasant behavior on the part of family members. Instilling courtesy, understanding, and tactful ways of responding to upset families should be part of the training of all staff who have direct contact with patients and families.

## Conclusions

A system that saves or prolongs lives only to cast patients and families into the abyss of fragmented chronic care and financial and emotional ruin, while at the same time criticizing them for being "too emotional," is unjust. Many families are willing to make enormous sacrifices, but martyrdom is not a good basis for health care policy or practice. When families are pushed beyond their limits, the patient's care is jeopardized, the caregiver's health is at risk, professionals are frustrated, and the health care system is burdened by greater costs.

Our recommendations focus on human relationships, not technology. In our technology-driven, efficiency-oriented health care system, the simplest interventions are often the hardest to initiate. Implementing the recommendations outlined here will require training—in some cases, retraining—staff at all levels and will also call on the most precious of resources: time. Lest this time be considered wasted, it is important to weigh against this investment the time already spent in fruitless and frustrating confrontations with aggrieved and uncooperative family members. A health care system that depends so heavily on the patient care and management provided by families should involve families as partners rather than define them as problems.

## References

Almagor RC. 1996. Patients' right to die in dignity and the role of their beloved people. *Annual Review of Law and Ethics.* Berlin: Duncker & Humblot.

Beckman HB, KM Markakis, AL Suchman, and RM Frankel. 1994. The doctor-patient relationship and malpractice: Lessons from plaintiff depositions. *Archives of Internal Medicine* 154(12): 1365-70.

Butler DJ, RL Holloway, and M Gottlieb. 1998. Predicting resident confidence to lead family meetings. *Family Medicine* 30(5): 356-61.

Collopy B, N Dubler, and C Zuckerman. 1990. The ethics of home care: Autonomy and accommodation. *Hastings Center Report* 20(2): S1-16.

Dill AE. 1995. The ethics of discharge planning for older adults: An ethnographic analysis. *Social Science & Medicine* 41(9): 1289-99.

Dubler NN. 1995. The doctor-proxy relationship: The neglected connection. *Kennedy Institute of Ethics Journal* 5(4): 289-306.

Hickson GB, EW Clayton, SS Entman, CS Miller, PB Githens, K Whetten-Goldstein, and FA Sloan. 1994. Obstetricians' prior malpractice experience and patients' satisfaction with care. *Journal of the American Medical Association* 272(20): 1583-7.

Kuczewski MG. 1996. Reconceiving the family. The process of consent in medical decisionmaking. *Hastings Center Report* 26(2): 30-7.

Levine C. 1998. *Rough crossings: Family caregivers' odysseys through the health care system.* New York: United Hospital Fund.

Pearlman RA, RF Uhlmann, and NS Jecker. 1992. Spousal understanding of patient quality of life: Implications for surrogate decisions. *Journal of Clinical Ethics* 3(2): 114-21.

Pletcher LC and AG Deal. 1993. Parent-professional partnerships: Common misconceptions. *Family Enablement Messenger.*

Seckler AB, DE Meier, M Mulvihill, BE Paris. 1991. Substituted judgment: How accurate are proxy predictions? *Annals of Internal Medicine* 115(2): 92-8.

Siegler M. 1982. The physician-patient accommodation: A central event in clinical medicine. *Archives of Internal Medicine* 142(10): 1899-902.

Sulmasy DP, PB Terry, CS Weisman, DJ Miller, RY Stallings, MA Vettese, and KB Haller. 1998. The accuracy of substituted judgments in patients with terminal diagnoses. *Annals of Internal Medicine* 128(8): 621-9.

Tomlinson T, K Howe, M Notman, and D Rossmiller. 1990. An empirical study of proxy consent for elderly persons. *Gerontologist* 30(1): 54-64.

Zuckerman C. 1999. *End-of-life care decisions and hospital legal counsel: Current involvement and opportunities for the future.* New York: Milbank Memorial Fund, 8.

Zweibel NR and CK Cassel. 1989. Treatment choices at the end of life: A comparison of decisions by older patients and their physician-selected proxies. *Gerontologist* 29(5): 615-21.

# 15   'Til Death Do Us Part: Family Caregiving at the End of Life

*Connie Zuckerman*

Death is perhaps the one common bond that all of us share in life. While the sudden, traumatic death of a loved one brings unspeakable sorrow to families, in this age of technological and pharmaceutical advances more of us can expect that our loved ones will instead experience gradual deterioration and decline through chronic illnesses that eventually lead to death. For those family members providing hands-on care, as evidenced throughout this book, the demands of chronic illness and disability can be overwhelming. As a loved one nears death, however, many of these burdens can become even more intense. Family members become "the untrained, untutored carers who so willingly shoulder immense responsibilities, doing something they have never done before, every action, every day colored by the knowledge that soon they will lose the one they love" (Doyle 1994).

Family members caring for a loved one at the end of life often experience a series of difficult and frightening events. The physical needs of dying patients can be tremendous, placing extraordinary burdens on caregivers, some of whom have already provided years of care. Moreover, the body can often be sustained well beyond the mind, leaving loved ones physically present and dependent, though cognition and spirit have slipped away. Compounding the burden, health care professionals seldom prepare caregivers for what to expect when someone is dying, leaving many caregivers anxious, uncertain, and frightened about what they can generally expect and what constitutes suffering that can be alleviated with appropriate care and medication.

Few caregivers have a choice about whether or not to take on such daunting responsibilities. We can do little to control the forces of nature or fate; for most of us, the ties of intimacy and family propel us into the caregiving arena, no matter what else is happening in our lives. Impending death is a stimulus that brings families together, often in mutual support but sometimes to reopen old wounds and relive old grievances. Family members often need to work hard to mend strained relationships, bring closure to the past, and create memories to sustain them after the loved one is gone. It can be difficult and demanding, even if ultimately rewarding. Most dying patients worry about the strain on their family members. In one recent study of patients with life-threatening and life-limiting illnesses, patients identified the burden on their loved ones of their dying as one of their most important concerns (Singer, Martin, and Kelner 1999).

In addition to increased caregiving and emotional burdens, family caregivers and patients must contend with crucial decisions about care at the end of life. While various advance-directive mechanisms exist, allowing patients' wishes about end-of-life care to be respected beyond their ability to make decisions, for a variety of reasons health care professionals do not always inquire about their existence or incorporate them into patients' care (Dubler 1999). Communication between patients and their family members about their wishes for end-of-life treatment also sometimes falters, leaving family members uncertain about what decisions to make for their dying loved ones.

It is clear that family caregivers of dying patients find themselves in the most vulnerable and fragile positions they have probably ever occupied, with a level of physical exertion and emotional endurance probably unrivaled by any other experience they are likely to encounter. At a time when family caregivers have the greatest needs, the deficiencies in the health care system become ever more apparent. Health care institutions and professionals can and must improve their efforts to provide support and guidance to ease family caregivers' anxieties, reduce their physical burdens, and facilitate the decision-making process for end-of-life care.

## Physical, Emotional, and Financial Tolls at the End of Life

Surveys of family members present at their loved ones' end of life report an array of demanding caregiving tasks and responsibilities, given the severe symptoms and dependence such patients usually have as death approaches. The anguish of watching a loved one suffer, and feeling helpless to respond in any meaningful way, is a common experience for many family caregivers. Despite the modern advent of sophisticated pain and symptom management, too many patients still die in pain and discomfort (SUPPORT Principal Investigators 1995), a far cry from the peaceful, dignified death most people desire. In one study, families reported that they observed in their dying loved ones the presence of severe pain, dyspnea (labored breathing), fatigue, and confusion for at least half the time at moderate or extreme severity (Lynn et al. 1997). Such symptoms are difficult enough to witness and accept when a loved one is being cared for in a hospital or nursing home, but they are even harder to tolerate when a family member herself is trying to provide the hands-on care at home.

Many persons envision an ideal death taking place in the comfort of their own bed, surrounded by friends and family, but the demands this ideal places on involved family members is hard to overestimate. Many family members report that they experience severe anxiety at the thought of physically managing the dying process of their loved one. As one family member candidly admitted, "I was petrified of being responsible for her if she were sent home. I would have been scared to leave her alone for a moment in case she suffered another breathing attack" (Shulman 1995). Such vigilance means that fatigue and exhaustion inevitably accompany caring for dying family members at home, and many families do not receive the support and guidance from health care professionals that they need to endure the inordinate physical demands of this kind of caregiving. While families that receive assistance from programs such as hospice are often relieved of, or supported in, these physical caregiving responsibilities, these family members, who are considered to be part of the "unit of care" along with the patient, are still required to provide a significant amount of care until the patient's death.

Because a majority of deaths still occur in hospitals or long-term care facilities, few families see death managed in a way that primarily emphasizes the comfort and quality of life of the dying person. In these settings, families often receive little information about what is a part of the normal process of dying and what constitutes unnecessary suffering that can be relieved with proper attention or medication. Lack of familiarity with the signs and symptoms of death and with the basic bodily functions that gradually shut down as the body begins to die can lead to enormous anxiety on the part of family members. One caregiving husband wrote to his wife's physician after her death: "[We] needed to know how the disease would progress. We needed to know what the symptoms would be. We needed you to paint a picture for us, give us a sort of scenario about what we might expect to happen" (Gordon 1998). Few families receive such a portrait, nor even realize that they should inquire about its availability.

Numerous studies and surveys have confirmed that doctors themselves are often ill-equipped to communicate with patients and their loved ones about end-of-life care and treatment options, and are often unable to support patients and their families once the battle to cure appears to have been lost. As the previously cited letter continued, "It was quite obvious that the radiation treatment had failed . . . but you stood your distance as you talked. And, in fact, you rather shortly dismissed us from the consultation. . . . Donna's comment to me was that it was harder for you to talk about the test results than it was for us to hear them" (Gordon 1998).

Many physicians never receive training on how to support patients and communicate with their families through the dying process. Some carry the same fears and inhibitions in talking about death that are prevalent in the general population. Some take the fact of a patient's pending death as a sign of personal defeat or failure. Whatever the reason, the fact that all too often family caregivers feel woefully unprepared to handle their end-of-life caregiving responsibilities effectively is at least partly attributable to this lack of support and assistance from physicians.

The tasks of such physical caregiving may be more difficult because of the emotional trials that accompany the dying process. Families may struggle with an array of conflicting and competing emotions, some anchored deeply in a lifetime of familial turmoil, and some as a result of the anticipatory grieving that naturally accompanies the impending loss of a loved one. It is common for family caregivers to experience guilt and concern about whether they are doing enough and about their own exhaustion, which ultimately limits their caregiving stamina. Many feel angry that caregiving sweeps aside other aspects of their lives, and harbor shame about secretly desiring the end to arrive.

The burden on family members may be enormous, not only because of the inevitable death of the loved one, but also because of the physical toll the care takes on them. As the philosopher Daniel Callahan stated, "The concern is when the care begins to destroy the caretaker" (Stewart 1997). Family caregivers often experience greater illness due to their caregiving responsibilities, especially because many are older and suffer from chronic, debilitating conditions themselves. One recent study suggests that the mental and emotional strain of caregiving is itself an independent risk factor for death among elderly caregiving spouses (Schulz and Beach 1999).

Fiscally, as well, many caregivers suffer enormous repercussions in the face of their loved one's terminal illness. Whether it is the actual expenditure of money for care not reimbursed by insurance, or the lost salaries or resources foregone as a result of needing to be present for a dying loved one, many families find themselves both emotionally and fiscally stressed (see Chapter 12, "The Financial Impact of Caregiving"). One study demonstrated that many families lose most of their savings or their major source of income as a result of caregiving at the end of life (Covinsky et al. 1994). While most family members willingly and lovingly provide such care, it can clearly take a tremendous toll on everyone involved.

## Advance Directives: Mechanisms and Mishaps

While new medical technologies and treatments can now prolong the lives of those facing serious and even life-threatening illnesses, the quality of life under such circumstances can often be severely diminished. Many individuals die months, sometimes years, after their cognitive capacity has declined. In fact, to the family members of such patients, their actual death is a haunting epilogue to the loss of their loved ones as they knew them, sometimes years before. This is especially true of patients who suffer from such debilitating conditions as Parkinson's disease, Alzheimer's disease, or other dementias.

Beginning in the 1960s, various legal mechanisms began to be developed to empower individual patients to make decisions about end-of-life treatments. Through judicial cases and legislative actions, these mechanisms, grouped under the concept of "advance directives," gave family members the legal authority to carry out these wishes should their loved ones lose decisional capacity. The most common of these mechanisms are the health care proxy, the living will, and the "do not resuscitate" (DNR) order.

### Health Care Proxies and Living Wills

The health care proxy—also known as the health care power of attorney or the durable power of attorney for health care decisions—and the living will are the most broadly applicable and utilized advance directives. These legal devices exist in some form in every state, though the requirements of language and execution and limitations on the applicability of such mechanisms may differ from one state to another. While in many circumstances documents filled out in one state will be honored and respected even if the patient winds up receiving care in a different state, there is never a guarantee of such, and patients and their families must be aware of their own state's requirements to ensure respect of their wishes wherever care is likely to be delivered. (For some patients who travel back and forth between certain states in the winter and summer months, it is wise to fill out separate documents to meet the specific requirements of each state.)

The health care proxy or health care power of attorney is perhaps the most valuable advance directive. With such an appointment, patients empower a chosen substitute, most often a close family member or loved one, to make decisions on their behalf, when and if they no longer have decision-making capacity. In fact, under such arrangements, patients may legally hand over to their proxies the authority to make the same type and breadth of decisions that they could still make for themselves, including decisions to withhold or withdraw life-prolonging measures.

In ideal circumstances, when patients transfer such authority they have implicit trust and confidence in the judgment and decisions of the appointed proxy. Such trust and confidence not only exist in the relationship between the patient and the proxy but are also solidified by clear communication about the values and choices the patient wishes to guide any surrogate decision making. This allows the patient to ensure that her choices are clearly understood, and provides the opportunity for the proxy to better understand the nature of the proxy responsibility, and whether to accept such an appointment in the first place.

All too often, however, such explicit discussions between patients and their chosen proxies never occur. Some proxies first learn of their appointment when they receive a phone call in the middle of the night about their loved one's sudden loss of capacity, or realize their discomfort or inability to fulfill the role they accepted when they are confronted with the actual decisions at hand. Such late discoveries serve the interests of neither the patient nor the surrogate decision maker. Yet they happen all too frequently, especially when physicians join this conspiracy of silence by not inquiring about the patient's execution of an advance directive well before a crisis occurs.

Family members who serve as surrogate decision makers, either through appointment as proxies or less formally in their roles as next of kin, must juggle the tremendous weight of these difficult decisions, often in an alien and not always friendly institutional environment. They must come to terms with their own emotions while trying to learn, as quickly as possible, hospital protocols and the expected course of their loved one's disease. While family members do their best, and sometimes fall short, health care professionals often view them as troublesome and inappropriate (Levine and Zuckerman 1999). It is hard to listen carefully when one's mind is preoccupied, when one doesn't know what to listen for, or when one's own words or concerns are not being heard. Unfortunately, not all care providers have the sensitivity or tolerance to recognize that to serve the interests of the patient, one must often respond to the needs of the surrogates as well.

For some patient and family constellations, this notion of autonomous decision making for patients, and transfer of decisional authority to a surrogate, may directly contradict familial patterns or dynamics of decision making on important matters. In some circumstances, cultural values do not even permit discussion of death and dying with the ill loved one. While the notion of individual autonomy is the core foundation for Western philosophic approaches to self-governance and decision making, many non-Western cultures and their adherents who reside in Western societies do not share this outlook. For such families the struggle to be understood and to do right by one's relative may be all the more challenging, and all the less possible.

In theory, health care providers are obligated to respect the choices of the health care proxy in the same manner in which they would respect the patient's own decisions. The reality of the clinical implementation of such transferred authority, however, is rarely so clear and decisive. It is not uncommon for health care professionals to challenge the decisions of appointed health care proxies. In some instances health care professionals confront proxies at a critical moment, advising that a particular intervention be made to save the patient's life, even when it is clear that the patient does not desire such an intervention. This places health care proxies in the dually excruciating circumstance of fighting for the decision-making authority with which they have already been legally vested, and then allowing their loved one to die. Sometimes proxies themselves, despite their knowledge of the wishes of their loved ones, cannot bring themselves to advocate for, or insist upon, decisions that would quicken the dying process. For many reasons, then, proxies often find themselves in deeply ambiguous and troubling roles.

A living will is usually a written document that articulates the patient's wishes regarding the use, withholding, or withdrawal of life-prolonging measures. While usually associated with forgoing or stopping such treatments, the living will is actually a vehicle for patients to declare their wishes, whatever they may be, including a desire for continued or attempted life-sustaining interventions, even if the prognosis is dismal or the condition severe. While some states require the living will to conform to a specific form, or to contain specific language, other states allow for more flexibility in the description of wishes and the implementation of the declaration. In some states, even an "oral advance directive" can be respected. Such a directive exists when the patient, prior to loss of capacity, has clearly articulated her choices and treatment values, although such decisions never actually made their way to being documented in any formal or informal manner.

For some patients, a living will provides peace of mind that their wishes will be clearly followed and the burden of decision making will be removed from their loved ones. Family members often appreciate having such a document as an authoritative guide to ensuring that their loved one's wishes are respected, and as a way to make sense of the often traumatic decision-making responsibility they have inherited. For some patients, however, there are no loved ones to rely upon at the moment of crisis, and they must look to the living will as the best method to help ensure that their values and priorities are respected beyond their ability to speak for themselves.

But living wills are not foolproof, and the extent of respect and authority they command can be as thin as the paper on which they are written. That is, the document must surface, make its way to the medical chart, and be pertinent and relevant to the specific situation at hand for it to impose its full breadth of authority. Some documents never make their way out of locked drawers at home or bank safe-deposit boxes, and thus have no impact on end-of-life decisions. Others are never brought forth because hospitals, nursing homes, or other care providers fail to inquire about their existence, despite the federal law that requires all health care providers to make such inquiries (Patient Self-Determination Act 1991). It is easy for inquiry regarding such documents to slip between the cracks, particularly when hospital admissions occur under stressful circumstances or busy hospital units mean less careful attention from health care professionals. As one involved daughter described her experience, "Exactly the opposite of what [my mother] had wished had occurred; the living will had become invisible just when it was needed most. My mother's physician, it turned out, had not notified the medical team of her advance directive, and the hospital . . . did not ask my mother whether she had such a document" (Hansot 1996). Having a living will, therefore, is no guarantee of its respect or relevance, and implementing its directives may require vigilance and advocacy on the part of fragile and vulnerable patients and their loved ones, qualities few can muster in the face of serious illness and decline.

## Do Not Resuscitate Orders

Perhaps the most common, yet most narrowly focused, advance directive is the DNR order. The need for such an order arises when there is a question as to whether to attempt cardiopulmonary resuscitation (CPR) when a patient's heart stops beating or lungs stop breathing. Such events typically occur as the body is in its last stages of the dying process, though they can occur for other reasons prior to death. In certain conditions, attempts to halt or reverse the process can forestall death, at least for a short period of time. The implementation of CPR, however, can involve desperate and traumatic interventions, including open heart massage, breaking of chest bones to push air in and out of lungs, or connecting the patient to a respirator, a mechanical breathing device on which seriously ill patients often become permanently dependent. For the very elderly and debilitated, and terminally ill patients, such efforts at CPR usually fail; the majority of such patients who are resuscitated do not survive to be discharged from the hospital.

For many patients, the possibility of undergoing CPR is considered just one more assault on the body in the dying process, and they want nothing to do with it. In such cases, the patient herself can request that a DNR order be placed on her medical chart, so that doctors will know not to perform CPR as the likelihood of death becomes clearer. Many patients, however, do not know about DNR orders, or are not given the opportunity to consider such a decision before their loss of capacity. As a result, when the patient loses decision-making capacity and death appears near, a family member will often be approached to decide whether to institute a DNR order for the patient. In fact, studies indicate that 70 percent to 93 percent of incapacitated patients with DNR orders obtained them through decisions made by their family members after the patients' loss of decisional capacity (Tilden et al. 1995).

In many institutional settings, participating in the DNR decision has become something of a rite of passage on the way toward a loved one's death. Some family members are relieved to have the opportunity to ensure that such futile and painful interventions are not performed on their loved one as the final moments approach, and they are often comforted by the belief that he or she would have been in agreement with this decision. For other family members, agreeing to a DNR order and signing a consent form for it are unbearable acts that cast a sense of guilt and responsibility on them, as though the act of signing such a consent form consigns the patient to a certain death that would otherwise not occur. Some family members, regardless of what they know (or don't know) about the patient's own wishes, will insist on CPR as a way to keep hope alive and perhaps forestall death, even in the face of almost certain failure. Such situations often occur when there has been a breakdown in communication between family and professional caregivers about the goals of care and what is realistically possible for the patient. But sometimes families are responding based on concerns that health care professionals might abandon their loved ones as death approaches. While DNR orders theoretically apply only to the narrow circumstance of a cardiopulmonary arrest, the all-too-frequent reality experienced by many families is that the DNR order ultimately becomes shorthand for "do not treat" or "do not care" attitudes on the part of overburdened and busy hospital professionals. Family members may not always fully realize or admit the burdens imposed by CPR on many seriously ill patients, but they surely understand the need to ensure that their loved ones are not abandoned by health care professionals as life draws to a close.

## Advance Directives: Common, but Not Ubiquitous

The need for an advance directive, and its use in clinical care delivery, is now a regular occurrence in end-of-life care. In fact, with modern medical technology, the majority of deaths are "orchestrated"—that is, purposeful decisions are made to withhold or withdraw life-sustaining interventions, leading to the death of the patient, usually after the patient has permanently lost decision-making capacity. Surveys show that most individuals want their family members to make end-of-life decisions for them if they lose the capacity to make such decisions on their own (Tilden et al. 1995). In fact, one study estimates that as many as 86 percent of all decisions about continuing life support involve substitute decision makers (Swigart et al. 1996), and the overwhelming majority are likely to be the intimate others and loved ones of the patients.

Some patients, however, purposefully do not appoint a loved one as health care proxy because they do not want to burden that person with such enormous responsibility. Others choose not to appoint a family member as proxy because they believe that person will be too overwhelmed with his or her own grief to be able to make decisions. Still others determine that their loved ones do not share their views and values on end-of-life decisions, and pick another person to be the proxy.

Despite educational and advocacy efforts by professional and consumer organizations, far too many people still do not consider and discuss end-of-life treatment options and wishes before a life-threatening illness strikes. For most people, the natural inhibition about pondering one's own mortality prevents them from planning for this inevitability, even if they know conceptually just how hard it will be for their loved ones to assume this task in their place. It is difficult to make and carry out such decisions even if one knows exactly what the patient would have wanted. That decisional responsibility becomes all the more haunting and anxiety provoking when the patient's wishes are unknown.

## Opportunities for Improvement

The portrait that emerges of family caregiving at the end of life is one characterized by difficulty, uncertainty, and a frequent lack of support from the health care system. All of the tensions, traumas, frustration, and loneliness that often accompany family caregiving of the ill and disabled (Levine 1999) can be intensified and exacerbated by the pending death of a loved one. It is incumbent upon health care professionals who have knowledge and expertise about the dying process to ease these burdens on family caregivers. There is even the potential that family caregivers may find this to be a deeply rewarding experience, provided they have the level of support necessary to ease the physical and emotional hardships of their caregiving activities.

Many family caregivers who have weathered the process have made helpful, often simple, suggestions for ways that health care professionals can help. One woman, whose mother died suddenly and unexpectedly when she left the bedside for just a moment, was never informed by her mother's health care team that her mother was dying. Wanting to ensure that no others find out as she did, she offers the following suggestions:

- Each patient's chart should have an area that is checked off when family members have been told that a patient is dying.
- Doctors should ask family members if they would like to be present when their loved one is dying.
- Doctors should provide family members with a list of signs that death is approaching (Taylor 1997).

Some researchers have gathered other suggestions from family caregivers about ways that health care institutions can ease the burdens on family members providing care for a dying loved one (Jacobson et al. 1997). These caregivers suggest that health care institutions should:

- Provide a checklist for families with specific guidance about necessary activities after death.
- Provide better referrals to support groups.
- Modify policies to ensure expanded visitation opportunities for dying patients and their loved ones.
- Train medical staff about ways to sensitively communicate with families about advance directives and ensure their full implementation.
- Screen employees for their capacity to be sensitive and caring to patients and their families.

Health care professionals can help families and health care proxies by discussing the signs and symptoms that will surface as the end of life approaches. No family should be left wondering, or belabored with unanswered questions, regarding the symptoms to anticipate and appropriate actions in response. No question is too trivial or too irrelevant at the end of a loved one's life.

It is imperative that health care professionals recognize that the physical burdens and emotional demands on family caregivers are often the most intense when patients are at the end of life. Within the resources that institutions and families have available, efforts must be made to increase assistance to family caregivers, whether that entails making early referrals to hospice or respite programs, advocating for increased nursing coverage when a patient is discharged, or simply making patient rooms more comfortable for family members who are spending extended periods at the bedside. Drawing from suggestions made by other family caregivers (Levine 1998), health care professionals must provide family caregivers with appropriate, comprehensive training to perform the necessary tasks at home, as these tasks become even more complicated, urgent, and anxiety provoking when a patient is at the end of life. Additionally, health care institutions should provide a phone number for caregivers to call at any time to reach a professional who is knowledgeable and can answer their questions.

Families can also make the process easier on themselves by openly and candidly discussing treatment choices and values that the patient wishes to be respected at the end of life. Patients and families should initiate this dialogue well before the onset of an illness or trauma that could impair decision making. In every community, hospice programs, advocacy groups, and consumer organizations have literature and trained counselors to help facilitate such discussions. At the same time, health care professionals can assist by encouraging families to begin such discussions, if they are congruent with the family's values and beliefs.

Many of these suggestions rest on the need for robust and timely communication between patients and their loved ones, patients and their providers, and providers and the family caregivers who are present at the end of life. Active planning, active listening, and engaged collaboration are the essential ingredients for professionals and intimates to ensure a peaceful passing for a dying loved one. While not all family members may be able or willing to take on such a task, for those who do our utmost support must be at hand.

### References

Covinsky KE, L Goldman, EF Cook, R Oye, N Desbiens, D Reding, W Fulkerson, AF Connors, Jr., J Lynn, and RS Phillips. 1994. The impact of serious illness on patients' families. SUPPORT investigators. Study to understand prognoses and preferences for outcomes and risks of treatment. *Journal of the American Medical Association* 272(23): 1839-44.

Doyle D. 1994. *Caring for a dying relative.* Oxford: Oxford University Press.

Dubler NN, ed. 1999. Symposium: The doctor-proxy relationship. *Journal of Law, Medicine & Ethics* 27(1): 5-86.

Gordon S. 1998. Letter to a patient's doctor. *Annals of Internal Medicine* 129(4): 333-4.

Hansot E. 1996. A letter from a patient's daughter. *Annals of Internal Medicine* 125(2): 149-51.

Jacobson JA, LP Francis, MP Battin, GJ Green, C Grammes, J VanRiper, and J. Gully. 1997. Dialogue to action: Lessons learned from some family members of deceased patients at an interactive program in seven Utah hospitals. *Journal of Clinical Ethics* 8(4): 359-71.

Levine C. 1998. *Rough crossings: Family caregivers' odysseys through the health care system.* New York: United Hospital Fund.

————. 1999. The loneliness of the long-term caregiver. *New England Journal of Medicine* 340(20): 1587-90.

Levine C and C Zuckerman. 1999. The trouble with families: Toward an ethic of accommodation. *Annals of Internal Medicine* 130(2): 148-52.

Lynn J, JM Teno, RS Phillips, AW Wu, N Desbiens, J Harrold, MT Claessens, N Wenger, B Kreling, and AF Connors, Jr. 1997. Perceptions by family members of the dying experience of older and seriously ill patients. *Annals of Internal Medicine* 126(2): 97-106.

Patient Self-Determination Act, Omnibus Budget Reconciliation Act of 1990, Pub. L. 101-508 Section 4206,475 1(OBRA), 42 USC Section 1395 cc ( f) (1) & 42 USC Section 1396 a (a) (Supp. 1991).

Schulz R and SR Beach. 1999. Caregiving as a risk factor for mortality: The Caregiver Health Effects Study. *Journal of the American Medical Association* 282(23): 2215-19.

Shulman B. 1995. A tolerable death. *Palliative Medicine* 9(4): 339-40.

Singer PA, DK Martin, and M Kelner. 1999. Quality end-of-life care: Patients' perspectives. *Journal of the American Medical Association* 281(2): 163-8.

Stewart B. 1997. Final days at home. *New York Times,* March 23, sec 13NJ, 1.

SUPPORT Principal Investigators. 1995. A controlled trial to improve care for seriously ill hospitalized patients. The study to understand prognoses and preferences for outcomes and risks of treatment (SUPPORT). *Journal of the American Medical Association* 274(20): 1591-8.

Swigart V, C Lidz, V Butterworth, and R Arnold. 1996. Letting go: Family willingness to forgo life support. *Heart & Lung* 25(6): 483-94.

Taylor D. 1997. On dying: Why was I not told? *Journal of Palliative Care* 13(4): 53-4.

Tilden VP, SW Tolle, MJ Garland, and CA Nelson. 1995. Decisions about life-sustaining treatment: Impact of physicians' behavior on the family. *Archives of Internal Medicine* 155(6): 633-8.

PART III

# *Responding to Caregivers' Needs*

# 16  Caregiving on the Public Policy Agenda

*Lynn Friss Feinberg*

The concept of caregiver support has emerged as a salient public policy issue. Policymakers are beginning to recognize the critical role families play in the provision of long-term care, and are addressing family-related matters that historically were thought to be too private for a public response (Feinberg 1997). As McConnell and Riggs point out, "If it is important to us as a society—as a matter of values or as a matter of resources—to maintain families as primary caregivers for people needing long-term care, then public policies that support those caregivers become even more important" (1994, 27).

For many public officials and decision makers, the impetus is their own experience of providing care to older parents, spouses, other relatives, or friends, or their knowing someone else who is a family caregiver. That trend will accelerate with the aging of the baby boom generation. By the year 2005, baby boomers will make up a majority of those 50 to 74 years of age, bringing with them an understanding of and concern with today's family issues, including caregiving (Russell 1995). Their influence in the public debate on caregiver support policies will only continue to grow.

The federal and state governments have strong incentives for supporting family caregiving:

- Most people who need long-term care prefer to receive assistance and services at home and to stay in their communities, near family and friends, for as long as possible. Indeed, informal care, particularly by the family, is the most important source of care for most older people.
- Families, not institutions or service providers, provide most long-

term care services. Virtually all older people living in non-institution-alized settings (about 95 percent of the total) receive at least some assistance from relatives and friends. About two out of three older persons living in the community (67 percent) rely solely on informal help, mainly from wives and adult daughters (Stone 2000).

• Families have long been filling the serious gaps in the long-term care system, such as the shortage of direct-care workers.

Despite increased recognition of family caregiving as a public policy is-sue, explicit support for family care continues to be highly variable in the United States. The lack of a uniform or cohesive support system poses major barriers for caregivers attempting to find and use the help they need. Families and friends of those requiring long-term care—particular-ly middle-class families—often have to navigate through and coordinate several disparate financing and delivery systems (Anderson and Knick-man 2001).

This chapter presents an overview of federal and state public policies and initiatives on family caregiving, focusing on four areas: direct servic-es, both multifaceted programs and single-focus strategies such as respite care; consumer direction; tax incentives; and employer-based mecha-nisms such as family-leave policies. Also highlighted are emerging areas of debate in caregiver support policy, including the payment of families to provide care, Lifespan Respite, and the relative value of tax strategies to provide some financial relief. The chapter concludes by addressing re-maining gaps and issues for the future.

## Direct Services

Home- and community-based services can directly assist families in their day-to-day caregiving responsibilities. Family caregiver support services can reduce caregiver distress and improve coping skills so that families can continue to provide care.

The Older Americans Act Amendments of 2000 established the National Family Caregiver Support Program (NFCSP), the first federal law to acknowledge and support the service needs of families in their caregiv-ing role. The passage of the NFCSP stands as the most significant legisla-tive accomplishment to date on behalf of family caregivers (Fox-Grage, Coleman, and Blancato 2001). With its creation, caregivers are now recog-nized as clients in their own right. The NFCSP calls for all states, working in partnership with Area Agencies on Aging (AAAs) and local community service providers, to offer caregivers:

- Information about available services;
- Assistance in gaining access to supportive services;
- Individual counseling, support groups, and training to assist with decision making and problem solving related to the caregiving role;
- Respite care, to provide temporary relief from caregiver responsibilities; and
- Supplemental services, on a limited basis, to complement the care provided by caregivers.

Those who are eligible for NFCSP services include family caregivers of persons age 60 or older, and grandparents and other related caregivers of children not more than 18 years of age. The federal law requires states to give priority to persons in greatest social and economic need, particularly low-income and minority individuals, and to older individuals providing care and support to persons with mental retardation and related developmental disabilities.

Included in the NFCSP are a Native American Caregiver Support Program ( funded at about $5 million dollars in 2002) and grants to organizations across the country to develop innovative approaches to assist family and informal caregivers and conduct projects of national significance. In September 2002, $7 million dollars were awarded to 39 agencies to assist in the development of multifaceted systems of caregiver support.

Federally funded at $125 million in FY 2001, $141.5 million in FY 2002, and $155.2 million in FY 2003, the NFCSP is still in the early stages of development in states across the country. To date, states vary considerably in how they have designed their caregiver support services and integrated them into their home- and community-based service systems. Overall, preliminary analysis suggests that the NFCSP is filling a gap for low- to moderate-income family caregivers, even though the current funding level is too low to meet their multifaceted needs (Feinberg, Newman, and Van Steenberg 2002).

Although the federal government is playing an increasingly important role, states have led the way in designing and financing diverse strategies to support and sustain family caregivers (Feinberg and Pilisuk 1999). While such programs are relatively new in many states, primarily the result of the infusion of NFCSP funds into those states' budgets, in several states caregiver support has a long tradition. Some, notably California, New Jersey, and Pennsylvania, have developed separate programs and specific funding and services for family caregivers. Others, such as Wisconsin, have integrated caregiver support into an array of community-based services. The successful family caregiver programs in these four states were, in large part, models for the NFCSP.

Both California and Pennsylvania are examples of states offering multifaceted statewide family caregiver support programs:

- The California Caregiver Resource Center (CRC) System, established by law in 1984 and administered by the California Department of Mental Health, provides a wide range of support services for families and caregivers of adults with cognitive impairments (e.g., Alzheimer's disease, stroke, traumatic brain injury). Administered locally by eleven regional, nonprofit agencies, the CRCs offer a comprehensive and flexible package of services, including specialized information and assistance; in-home caregiver assessment; family consultation and care planning; individual, group, and family counseling; Internet decision support; in-person and online support groups; legal and financial consultations with attorneys; and education and training. The CRCs also offer families a wide range of respite options and up to $3,600 a year for respite assistance, delivered through a voucher program and permitting payment to other family members or friends for respite care they provide. A separate state contract funds a State-wide Resources Consultant (SRC) to operate an information clearinghouse; conduct education, training, and applied research; carry out program and policy development; maintain a statewide database on CRC clients; and provide technical assistance to CRC sites. With $11.7 million in state general funds for FY 2002, the CRCs served over 14,000 California family caregivers. Since passage of the federal NFC-SP, many California Area Agencies on Aging (AAAs) have contracted with the state-funded CRCs to expand the population of caregivers they serve (Feinberg, Newman, and Van Steenberg 2002).
- The Pennsylvania Family Caregiver Support Program (FCSP), established by law in 1990 and administered by the Pennsylvania Department of Aging through 52 local AAAs, assists family caregivers of functionally dependent adults age 60 or older or people of any age with chronic dementia. The FCSP provides assessment, care management, benefits counseling, caregiver counseling, training and education, and access to support groups. Each family tailors services to fit

its own needs. Limited to families with incomes less than 380 percent of poverty level, the program also provides, on average, a monthly reimbursement of $200 for respite services, durable goods, or medical supplies. AAAs may reimburse caregivers as much as $500 per month, as long as the caseload average doesn't exceed $300 per month. A one-time reimbursement of up to $2,000 for home modifications and assistive devices is also available. While caregivers are reimbursed for expenses, they cannot be paid for their provision of respite or other caregiving tasks. In FY 2002, Pennsylvania expended $9.3 million in state general revenues for the program and served over 8,000 caregivers. Federal funds, under the NFCSP ($6.9 million in FY 2002), have allowed Pennsylvania to supplement and expand access to the state-funded FCSP services (Feinberg, Newman, and Van Steenberg 2002).

## Respite Care

Respite is the service most typically provided by publicly funded state and local agencies. Respite care addresses one of the most pressing needs identified by families, namely, temporary relief to reduce the strain that caregivers experience day in and day out (Alzheimer's Association 1991; Feinberg and Kelly 1995). The concept of Lifespan Respite is taking hold at the state as well as federal level. Lifespan Respite is "a coordinated system of accessible, community-based respite care services for caregivers regardless of age, race, ethnicity, special need or situation" (National Respite Coalition 2002). Four states—Oklahoma, Oregon, Nebraska, and Wisconsin—have implemented Lifespan Respite programs, and numerous other states have created coalitions to advocate for this approach. The goal is to "make respite more accessible by giving one agency authority to integrate available funds, ensure coordination of care, control costs and identify gaps in services and funds" (Fox-Grage, Coleman, and Blancato 2001, 6).

Nebraska's Lifespan Respite Services Program, for example, serves individuals of any age who provide care for persons with any disease or disability, unable to care for themselves. In 1999, the legislature appropriated $500,000 for FY 2000 and FY 2001 to develop the program; in May 2000, the Nebraska Department of Health and Human Services, acting as the lead agency, initiated it. In 2001 an additional $1 million per year was appropriated for respite care. Six community-based programs throughout the state are charged with assessing specific community needs; they also conduct marketing to increase public awareness of the program, recruit direct-care workers, develop and conduct caregiver training for service providers or families, and conduct a self-evaluation of the program (Fox-Grage, Coleman, and Blancato 2001).

A federal initiative, the Lifespan Respite Care Act of 2003 (S538, HR1083), was reintroduced in the 108th Congress to authorize $90.5 million in funds, beginning in FY 2004, to develop and evaluate programs at the state and local levels; provide both planned and emergency respite-care services; train and recruit respite-care workers and volunteers; and offer training programs to help families make informed decisions about respite-care services. Under separate authority the act would also establish a National Resource Center on Lifespan Respite Care. The secretary of Health and Human Services would be required to ensure coordination of respite for family caregivers at the federal level.

Supporters of this concept argue that there is no single, coordinated federal family caregiver program to support the development or implementation of Lifespan Respite services nationwide. They argue that although the NFCSP includes respite care as a component of a multifaceted caregiver support system, it is an age-categorical program, largely restricted to family or informal caregivers of persons age 60 and older and, to a much lesser extent, older caregivers caring for grandchildren or adult children with disabilities. Further, numerous other federal programs continue to provide respite assistance for caregivers of individuals with specific disabilities or functional levels, or of specific ages, resulting in continued fragmentation and lack of accessible respite care (ARCH National Respite Network 1999). Opponents, on the other hand, believe that the newly created NFCSP serves as the infrastructure and should be used as the vehicle to expand and coordinate *all* caregiver support, including respite care.

The overall lack of consistency and coordination in states' programs is particularly frustrating to caregivers as they try to locate and negotiate a complex maze of services for their loved ones and themselves. Some states are working to improve service delivery to family caregivers. In Maryland, for example, a 2001 law (SB 567) created a Caregivers Support Coordinating Council, under the Department of Human Resources. The Council is charged with coordinating statewide planning, development, and implementation of family caregiver support services. Such coordinated state efforts are vitally important to address the wide range of caregiver support programs available in states with different eligibility requirements, divergent funding sources, and varied funding levels.

## Consumer Direction

A growing national "consumer direction" movement aims to give beneficiaries who are eligible for long-term care services more choice and control in arranging for personal assistance. An estimated 60 percent of state Medicaid programs offer some consumer direction and many other state-funded programs also provide this option (Fox-Grage, Coleman, and Blancato 2001). Rather than a single approach, consumer direction consists of a range of models that vary in terms of how much decision making, control, and autonomy are shifted from service providers to the consumers of services (Benjamin 2001). Under the NFCSP, states can offer caregivers a number of consumer-directed options, including supplemental services (e.g., assistive devices or consumable supplies), a variety of respite arrangements, and direct payments for respite care. As such, the NFCSP presents an opportunity to expand consumer-directed programs offering family and informal caregivers a chance to select goods or services that will benefit them *directly*, rather than indirectly through benefits to care recipients (Feinberg, Newman, and Van Steenberg 2002).

The national Cash and Counseling Demonstration and Evaluation, begun in October 1995, is a policy-driven study of a consumer-directed approach to personal assistance services for older people and younger adults with disabilities. Funded by the U.S. Department of Health and Human Services, Office of the Assistant Secretary for Planning and Evaluation, and The Robert Wood Johnson Foundation, this three-state (Arkansas, Florida, New Jersey) Medicaid demonstration tests the use of a cash benefit to enhance Medicaid consumers' ability to design services that best meet their needs. Consumers receive a monthly cash allowance to purchase goods and services, and counseling to help plan those purchases. They may purchase personal assistance from sources other than traditional Medicaid providers, such as family members or friends. Arkansas's early experiences show that about 78 percent of participants who chose the cash option hired paid caregivers who were family members (Brown and Foster 2000). A report on the lessons to be drawn from all three demonstration projects was released in 2003 (Phillips et al.). Due to the early success of the demonstrations, as well as interest from other states, The Robert Wood Johnson Foundation, the U.S. Department of Health and Human Services' Office of the Assistant Secretary for Planning and Administration, and the Administration on Aging have authorized an expansion of the program, with up to ten states expected to be awarded three-year grants in summer 2004 to implement the Cash and Counseling model.

Current Medicaid policy prohibits the direct provision of services benefiting the family or informal caregiver, and payment to spouses or to parents of minor children for the care they provide (Kaiser Commission on Medicaid and the Uninsured 2001). Yet Medicaid could better meet the needs of consumers by explicitly providing meaningful support services to family caregivers and allowing the consumer-directed option to pay families to provide care. Cash and Counseling could potentially help move Medicaid and other home- and community-based services programs toward just such a "family systems" approach.

Despite the critical role that families play in long-term care, the practice of paying families to provide care is controversial in the U.S. Supporters view such payments as an important consumer-directed option for people with disabilities and their families, increasing consumer choice and quality of care; placing a monetary value on the labor of family caregivers; expanding the limited direct-care worker supply; serving as a more cost-effective option than the usual agency-directed services; and appealing particularly to the next generation of elderly, the baby boomers (Polivka 2001; Simon-Rusinowitz, Mahoney, and Benjamin 1998). Critics, on the other hand, are concerned about poor quality of services, fraud and abuse, and fears of exploding public costs for services that have traditionally been provided for "free" by family and friends (Blaser 1998). Another argument points out that this option pays family members at very low rates, offers little or no "career advancement" and no benefits, and is simply a way to reduce costs of care. Critiques notwithstanding, there appears to be a growing interest in consumer-directed models that support families, as states look for options that increase consumer satisfaction without substantial new investments of public funds.

## Tax Incentives

The emotional and physical strain of caregiving is often exacerbated by worries over paying for care. Some caregiving spouses, for example, forgo hiring any help at home because they are anxious and concerned about how they will cover costly extended nursing home care if it becomes necessary. Tax deductions and tax credits are two strategies utilized by policy makers to provide some financial relief to caregivers.

Tax deductions tend to favor higher-income people, giving them more subsidy per dollar deducted than taxpayers in lower-income brackets (McConnell and Riggs 1994). Beginning in 1997, out-of-pocket expenses for long-term care, including custodial care and long-term care insurance premiums, could be deducted as medical expenses by those itemizing on their tax returns. Since fewer than 5 percent of taxpayers itemize their medical/dental claims, however, this deduction is available to very few (U.S. Department of Labor 2000a). Moreover, such deductions are of little use to the family caregiver who has quit a job to provide care (McConnell and Riggs 1994).

Unlike tax deductions, tax credits generally benefit lower-income taxpayers and are viewed as a fairer way of providing tax incentives for family caregivers. In recent years, tax credit legislation has gained more political appeal among some policy makers, though no federal law has been enacted to date. Several bills have been introduced in Congress over the past two years to give taxpayers credits of up to $3,000 if they need long-term care or if they provide long-term care for a spouse or dependent. Proponents generally view tax credits as a step toward improving federal long-term care policy and reducing the costs of care. Critics, on the other hand, say they don't go far enough in providing financial relief to caregivers or individuals with long-term care needs, particularly middle-income family members who are hardest hit and most at risk of bankruptcy. We can expect to see continued debate on this tax strategy in coming years.

Many states have enacted laws intended to provide financial relief for caregivers, in the form of either a tax deduction or tax credit. To date, 22 states and the District of Columbia provide tax breaks. Some states offer a deduction for expenses, usually up to $2,400, but most offer a credit instead (National Conference of State Legislatures 2000). In California, for instance, a modest $500 tax credit took effect on January 1, 2001, for taxpayers who require long-term care or provide long-term care to family members. These state tax credits are a small step toward providing very limited financial relief to caregivers.

### Employer-Based Mechanisms

The financial impact of caregiving is most apparent for family caregivers when it affects their ability to engage in and perform effectively at work (see Chapter 11, "Caregiving and the Workplace"). An estimated 25 percent of all workers provide elder care (Bond, Galinsky, and Swanberg 1998). Among working people caring for a family member or friend aged 65 or older, two-thirds report having to rearrange their work schedule, decrease their hours, or take an unpaid leave in order to meet their caregiving responsibilities (U.S. Department of Health and Human Services 1998). Many working caregivers cannot afford to take time off without receiving a paycheck, however.

The Family and Medical Leave Act (FMLA), enacted in 1993, was the first national legislation designed to offer some important protections to working people to help them fulfill both their work and family responsibilities, including family caregiving. It guarantees workers in businesses with at least 50 employees 12 weeks of unpaid leave each year to care for a newborn or newly adopted child or seriously ill family member, or to recover from their own serious health conditions, and a return to their jobs. According to the National Partnership for Women & Families (2002b), the FMLA has been a great success, allowing more than 35 million working family members to care for their loved ones without putting their jobs or their health insurance at risk.

But the FMLA offers only minimal support to people who are juggling work and family (Wagner 2001). Many employed caregivers—about 43 percent of the workforce—do not benefit from it at all, because they work for businesses with fewer than 50 employees (Holcomb 2002). Moreover, most employed caregivers cannot afford to take *unpaid* leave. The U.S. lags behind nearly every other industrialized nation in the world in terms of paid family leave. According to the U.S. Department of Labor (2000b), more than three in four employees (78 percent) who have needed but have not taken family or medical leave say they cannot afford to do so.

Although advocates have mounted a nationwide campaign to amend the FMLA, for the foreseeable future states will continue to take the lead in expanding and improving family leave benefits. A significant number of states (as well as the District of Columbia and Puerto Rico) have enacted their own versions of the FMLA that are more generous than the original (National Partnership for Women & Families 2002c). Federal FMLA provisions have been expanded in several ways: applying leave provisions to workers in companies with fewer than 50 employees (comprehensive leave laws in the District of Columbia, Oregon, and Vermont, and some coverage in 14 other states); allowing leave for family medical needs that are not covered by the federal law (Maine, Massachusetts, and Vermont); expanding the definition of "family" (District of Columbia, Hawaii, Oregon, Rhode Island, and Vermont); extending the time periods for family and medical leave (California, Connecticut, the District of Columbia, Louisiana, Oregon, Puerto Rico, Rhode Island, and Tennessee); and offering paid leave (California).

In September 2002, California became the first state in the nation to enact paid family leave. SB1661 entitles employees who take time off to care for a newborn, newly adopted child, or seriously ill family member up to six weeks of partially paid leave a year. Employees began paying into the program on January 1, 2004, and benefits became available beginning in July 2004. The program, funded entirely by payroll deductions, expands the state fund that now provides insurance for disabled workers. Although employees pay an average of only $27 per year, workers on leave will bring home 55-60 percent of their wages, up to $728 per week during the program's first year (National Partnership for Women & Families 2002a). Family-leave bills were pending in 26 other states in 2002, and 20 of those states held hearings on the topic (Prah 2002). Others will likely expand and improve family-leave benefits now that California has taken the first step to support paid leave.

Another promising strategy is the federal Long-Term Care Security Act. This legislation, along with the National Family Caregiver Support Program, was signed into law in November 2000 by President Clinton, as part of his long-term care initiative. The law established the Federal Long-Term Care Insurance Program, enabling federal employees, retirees, military personnel, and their spouses and other qualified relatives to purchase long-term care insurance at group rates (Newman 2002).

Several features of this new insurance program could be especially beneficial to caregivers. First, unlike most long-term care insurance programs, the federal program allows relatives of enrollees, as well as traditional care coordinators who are registered nurses, to provide care-coordination services themselves. This consumer-directed option is an important one for many family caregivers who are the primary care managers for their loved ones. Second, the program covers respite services and care provided in a range of settings: nursing home, assisted living facility, hospice, adult day care center, and home. Third, family members (other than those who lived in the home of the enrollee at the time she/he became eligible for benefits) can be paid to provide respite care at home, up to 365 days in an enrollee's lifetime (U.S. Office of Personnel Management 2002). Lastly, caregiver training is a covered benefit, enabling family members, friends, or neighbors to receive the hands-on skill training needed to provide quality care.

If a sufficiently high percentage of federal employees and military personnel enroll in long-term care insurance plans, states may consider similar programs on behalf of their employees (Fox-Grage, Coleman, and Blancato 2001) and include these caregiver support benefits. But while long-term care insurance can be useful for some families, it may be unaffordable for most or unavailable for those with pre-existing conditions. Despite growing efforts in the industry, and some incentives enacted at the state and federal levels, long-term care insurance pays for less than 7 percent of the nation's long-term care costs (Feder, Komisar, and Niefeld 2000).

## Issues for the Future

Recognizing and supporting family and friends who provide care is a critical component of a comprehensive long-term care system. Despite some recent reforms, explicit support for family caregiving continues to be highly variable in the U.S., with no cohesive or uniform caregiver support system. States differ widely in their approach to caregiver support with various direct services and other strategies (e.g., family leave, tax incentives) developed, oftentimes, in a piecemeal fashion. In particular, the fragmentation of services and policies leaves caregivers confused, overwhelmed, and facing major barriers to finding and using the help they need. At the national level, the modest funding for the NFCSP leaves gaps in caregiver support services that vary substantially from state to state as well as within states. All families should have access to at least a minimum level of explicit caregiver support services regardless of where they live. Increasing funds for the NFCSP will provide support for more caregivers and help to sustain them in their caregiving role, in turn reducing the fiscal pressures on Medicaid and other state-funded home- and community-based programs (Feinberg, Newman, and Van Steenberg 2002).

One of the major national long-term care policy developments in recent years came in June 1999 when the U.S. Supreme Court ruled in the landmark case *Olmstead v L.C.* that states were required to provide services to certain persons with disabilities in community settings rather than institutions. In essence *Olmstead* requires that states plan for and undertake two basic activities that could serve as blueprints for future long-term care reforms: (1) restructuring existing programs and services in order to promote community integration; and (2) establishing an individualized assessment process to design community services. While the full implications of *Olmstead* are as yet unclear, family involvement in both planning and implementation are central to creating community services for the elderly and younger persons with disabilities, and to providing support for family caregivers (Rosenbaum 2001; Feinberg, Newman, and Van Steenberg 2002; Fox-Grage, Coleman, and Blancato 2001). Moreover, as both the federal government and the states focus on long-term care reforms, including reducing reliance on nursing homes and strengthening integrated systems of home- and community-based services, the impact of these policy shifts on family caregivers must be considered. As Stone (2000, 73) asserts, "The long-term care system must be sensitive to the needs of the family as well as those of the person who needs long-term care."

The biggest gap in current public policy for American families, particularly the middle class, is the financing of our long-term care system, however. Individuals who need long-term care must pay out of pocket until they are impoverished, before they can get help through the means-tested Medicaid program; lower-income persons are likely to be eligible for a wider array of long-term care services and options than the middle-income are (Anderson and Knickman 2001). According to McConnell and Riggs (1994, 34), "The real way to support family caregivers is to provide financial protection through a social insurance program that ensures affordable access to quality long-term care, in the setting that is most appropriate for the person needing care and best meets family needs."

Today, family and friends bear most of the burden of accessing, coordinating, and providing long-term care at home and in the community, without the support necessary to sustain them in the caregiving role. As we look to the future, a critical challenge is to ensure that family support is an explicit objective of all federal and state long-term care policies and programs. We owe it to ourselves and our families.

## References

Alzheimer's Association. 1991. *Time out! The case for a national family caregiver support policy.* Washington, DC: Alzheimer's Association.

Anderson G and JR Knickman. 2001. Changing the chronic care system to meet people's needs. *Health Affairs (Millwood)* 20(6): 146-60.

ARCH National Respite Network. 1999. Finding federal funds for respite and crisis care programs. Factsheet No. 52. www.archrespite.org/archfs52.htm. Accessed August 14, 2003.

Benjamin AE. 2001. Consumer-directed services at home: A new model for persons with disabilities. *Health Affairs (Millwood)* 20(6): 80-95.

Blaser CJ. 1998. The case against paid family caregivers: Ethical and practical issues. *Generations* 22(3): 64-5.

Bond JT, E Galinsky, and JE Swanberg. 1998. *The 1997 National Study of the Changing Workforce.* New York: Families and Work Institute.

Brown R and L Foster. 2000. *Cash and counseling: Early experiences in Arkansas. Trends in consumer choice.* Issue Brief No. 1. Washington, DC: Mathematica Policy Research.

Feder J, HL Komisar, and M Niefeld. 2000. Long-term care in the United States: An overview. *Health Affairs (Millwood)* 19(3): 40-56.

Feinberg LF. 1997. *Options for supporting informal and family caregiving.* San Francisco: American Society on Aging.

Feinberg LF and KA Kelly. 1995. A well-deserved break: Respite programs offered by California's statewide system of Caregiver Resource Centers. *The Gerontologist* 35(5): 701-5.

Feinberg LF, SL Newman, and C Van Steenberg. 2002. *Family caregiver support: Policies, perceptions and practices in 10 states since passage of the National Family Caregiver Support Program.* San Francisco: Family Caregiver Alliance.

Feinberg LF and TL Pilisuk. 1999. *Survey of fifteen states' caregiver support programs.* San Francisco: Family Caregiver Alliance.

Fox-Grage W, B Coleman, and RB Blancato. 2001. *Federal and state policy in family caregiving: Recent victories but uncertain future.* San Francisco: Family Caregiver Alliance.

Holcomb G. 2002. *Why Americans need family leave benefits and how they can get them.* Washington, DC: National Partnership for Women & Families.

Kaiser Commission on Medicaid and the Uninsured. 2001. *Medicaid: A primer.* Washington, DC: Henry J. Kaiser Foundation.

McConnell S and JA Riggs. 1994. A public policy agenda: Supporting family caregiving. In Cantor MH, ed. *Family caregiving: Agenda for the future.* San Francisco: American Society on Aging.

National Conference of State Legislatures. 2000. Tax incentives for caregivers. NCSL Legisbrief 8(24).

National Partnership for Women & Families. 2002a. *National Partnership for Women & Families' Monthly Bulletin on Paid Leave.* www.nationalpartnership.org/Content.cfm?L1=6&L2=2.0&L3=1&BID=17 Accessed July 21, 2004.

———. 2002b. *National Partnership for Women & Families News.* www.nationalpartnership.org/Content.cfm?L1=8&L2=4&AID=4&NID=16 Accessed July 21, 2004.

———. 2002c. *State family leave laws that are more expansive than the federal family and medical leave act.* www.nationalpartnership.org/Content cfm?L1=202&TypeID=1&NewsItemID=259  Accessed July 21, 2004.

National Respite Coalition. 2002. Lifespan respite. www.archrespite.org/NRC-Lifespan.htm  Accessed July 21, 2004.

Newman S. 2002. *Insuring your future: What caregivers need to know about long-term care insurance.* San Francisco: National Center on Caregiving, Family Caregiver Alliance.

Phillips B, K Mahoney, L Simon-Rusinowitz, J Schore, S Barrett, W Ditto, T Reimers, P Doty. 2003. *Lessons from the implementation of Cash and Counseling in Arkansas, Florida, and New Jersey.* Princeton, NJ: Mathematica Policy Research. www.hhp.umd.edu/AGING/CCDemo/Products/Complete3state.pdf Accessed July 21, 2004.

Polivka L. 2001. *Paying family members to provide care: Policy considerations for states.* San Francisco: Family Caregiver Alliance.

Prah P. 2002. Momentum for paid family leave grows.
    www.stateline.org/stateline/?pa=story&sa=showStoryInfo&id=266153
    Accessed July 21, 2004.
Rosenbaum S. 2001. *Olmstead v. LC: Implications for family caregivers.* San Francisco: Family Caregiver Alliance.
Russell C. 1995. The baby boom turns 50. *American Demographics* 17: 22-33.
Simon-Rusinowitz L, KJ Mahoney, and AE Benjamin. 1998. Payments to families who provide care: An option that should be available. *Generations* 2(3): 69-75.
Stone R. 2000. *Long-term care for the elderly with disabilities: Current policy, emerging trends, and implications for the twenty-first century.* New York: Milbank Memorial Fund.
U.S. Department of Health and Human Services. 1998. *Informal caregiving: Compassion in action.* Washington, DC: U.S. Department of Health and Human Services.
U.S. Department of Labor. 2000a. *Advisory Council on Employee Welfare and Pension Benefit Plans: Report, findings, and recommendations of the Working Group on Long-Term Care.* Washington, DC: U.S. Department of Labor.
————. 2000b. *Balancing the needs of families and employers: Family and medical leave surveys.* Washington, DC: U.S. Department of Labor.
U.S. Office of Personnel Management. 2002. Federal long-term care insurance program.  www.opm.gov/insure/ltc/  Accessed July 21, 2004.
Wagner DL. 2001. *Enhancing state initiatives for working caregivers.* San Francisco: Family Caregiver Alliance.

# 17 The Visiting Doctors Program: Bringing Care Home

*Shoshanna Korn-Meyer, CSW, Lili Toborg, NP, and Jeremy Boal, MD*

"Momma can't get out," noted the chief complaint on the referral sheet. Gazing up the murky stairwell, stretching six flights to the roof, that diagnosis was inarguable. As medical professionals making home visits in New York City, we have become connoisseurs of the vagaries of elevators and stairs, doormen buildings, housing projects, crosstown traffic, and the best way to hail a taxi.

A home visit is a profoundly different experience from a clinic or hospital encounter. Rather than meeting a patient as she sits, wearing a backless hospital gown, in a nondescript examination room, we meet patients in their homes, surrounded by their personal belongings. Instead of an otoscope mounted on the wall, there are macramé owls, portraits of JFK abutting photos of grandchildren, and the other myriad bric-a-brac of a lifetime. This difference can be very meaningful in the development of a relationship between patient and provider.

On a recent visit, we met Davida Brown (like the other patients and family caregivers described in this chapter, not her real name). She is bedbound and no longer able to speak after suffering a severe stroke. Had she been brought to the clinic or emergency room for an exam, she would have arrived by ambulance, on a stretcher, wrapped in a white sheet—a blank canvas. Visiting her home, however, afforded us the opportunity to visualize her life history as told by the walls of her apartment, which were covered with plaques and awards commemorating her long career as a teacher and her commitment to her church. There were photographs of her with her church friends and colleagues, as well as pictures of her late husband and of her nieces and nephews standing proudly in their graduation gowns and wedding finery. Mrs. Brown spent her life dedicated to her career, church, and family, and her home bears witness to this devotion.

Although she has no children of her own, Mrs. Brown has two nieces who are very involved in her care. Being in her home, seeing the record of her life, one can understand her nieces' loyalty and love and their commitment to ensuring that she receives the best care possible. One can appreciate how meaningful it is for her to remain in her home for as long as possible, rather than spend her last years in a nursing home, stripped of her past.

## "Drop-Out" Patients

The Visiting Doctors program began at New York City's Mount Sinai Hospital in 1997 as a pilot project by medical residents concerned about patients' loss of continuity of care. The residents had noted, anecdotally, that many patients admitted to the hospital for acute care were lost to follow-up once discharged home. At the same time, many patients followed in the primary care clinic appeared to vanish from the system after years of care, leaving no trace. Over time it became more obvious that, after developing critical degrees of cognitive and/or functional impairment, patients were simply unable to maintain adequate contact with primary care services. This loss of access to care usually occurred at precisely the moment when they had the greatest need for care. It seemed reasonable to assume that the gap in services contributed to further declines in health status and led to poor outcomes for patients.

Large-scale, well-defined systems for addressing the ongoing needs of severely debilitated patients who wish to remain at home are few and far between. The general lack of coordination between service providers, the intermittent nature of service delivery, and the frequent need for emergency medical services contribute to a failure to meet basic and humane care standards. For example, Medicare-covered home health care services are designed to provide skilled nursing care and social work support in the home for specified periods of time after a discrete incident, such as a hospitalization or a change in general medical condition. While these services are of great benefit to patients upon discharge from acute inpatient hospital care, they are typically short-term, leaving homebound patients without sustained services.

This gap has forced legions of overwhelmed and underappreciated family members and friends to navigate the "system," with limited support, on behalf of their loved ones. As this book has amply demonstrated, the burden of caregiving would be challenging enough in a coordinated, well-oiled care system. Unfortunately, it is all the greater given the degree of fragmentation, poor communication, and lack of resources that most patients and caregivers face.

### Delivering Care—Literally

The Visiting Doctors program provides primary care in the home to over 600 men and women each year. The program's primary providers are four doctors and four nurse practitioners, all of whom make home visits to their panels of patients. A full-time social worker and a full-time Spanish-language translator are on staff as well. The physicians, nurse practitioners, and social worker meet three times each week to discuss challenging cases. Providers work closely with certified home health agencies, community-based social service agencies, and home hospice programs.

The nurse practitioners, who devote full time to the homebound program, make home visits every weekday morning; their afternoons are reserved for administrative work. Physician providers devote 50 percent of their time to the homebound program, making home visits three mornings per week and keeping two additional half days protected for administrative work. Both physicians and nurse practitioners spend a considerable amount of non-visit time communicating with patients, caregivers, and others. (The other 50 percent of the physicians' time is used in a variety of activities that include maintaining an outpatient practice in the hospitals' geriatrics and primary care clinics, teaching medical residents in the primary care clinic, attending on the inpatient wards and palliative care consult service, carrying out funded research projects, and performing other teaching activities.)

A full-time nurse is available in the office during regular business hours to triage patient problems over the phone. At night and on weekends, the program's eight providers rotate telephone on-call duty. A medical office assistant is responsible for ordering durable medical equipment, arranging for ancillary diagnostic testing (e.g., x-rays), stocking medical bags, and tracking blood drawn during home visits. Two administrative assistants are responsible for answering phones, submitting billing slips, and scheduling new and follow-up appointments.

The majority of patients served are frail, elderly men and women with limited financial resources. On average they are dependent in six of eight activities of daily living. Leading reasons for referral are dementia, stroke, frailty, psychiatric illness (including depression, anxiety, agoraphobia, and psychosis), severe heart failure, severe emphysema, and multiple sclerosis. While adults of all ages are cared for, the average patient age is 81; 88 percent of all patients are over age 65. The program serves clients throughout Manhattan, with the largest concentrations in the neighbor-hoods of East and West Harlem. Their ethnic breakdown reflects com-munity diversity: 42 percent of patients are white; 28 percent Latino; and 27 percent African American. Thirty-three percent live in public housing. The majority of patients have Medicare (90 percent), approximately half have Medicaid (55 percent), and 3 percent are uninsured. Three-quarters of our patients have family members and/or friends who assist with their care.

In addition to medical problems, the program's patients face complex non-medical issues that must be addressed in order to preserve and pro-mote health and well-being. These include poverty, caregiver burnout, non-continuous access to community-based social services, and elder abuse and neglect.

Over time, the Mount Sinai Visiting Doctors Program has drawn on its growing experience with family caregivers to better understand their needs, as well as those of patients who wish to remain at home. We now know that caregivers must be supported with the same intensity as our patients if we are to have a positive impact.

Our caregivers, too, are a very heterogeneous group, reflecting the wide variety of patients cared for by the program. Two-thirds of caregiv-ers are female. Ages range from 19 to 91 years, with a median of 56. Almost 80 percent of our caregivers are high school graduates, half are married, and 40 percent work full time. Almost half live with the patients they are caring for, and 57 percent have been providing care for at least five years.

As a group, they report extraordinary levels of burden related to care-giving. One-third feel that they are missing out on life, the same propor-tion wish they could escape their situation, and just over one-quarter have had adverse health consequences related to their caregiving respon-sibilities. Caregivers are more likely to have higher levels of burden when care recipients have more physical symptoms and/or lower levels of phys-ical functioning, are younger, or have never been married. Higher levels of caregiver burden are also associated with certain patient conditions, including dementia, depression, and a history of stroke.

Recent changes in Medicare reimbursement have helped to make our program and others like it financially viable. These changes include in-creased payments for physician and nurse practitioner home visits, pay-ment for oversight of the care plans of homebound patients receiving skilled nursing care in the home, and payment for certification of skilled nursing care. We have also received substantial financial support from our hospital system, which views our program as a mechanism for bringing patients into that system—generating inpatient admissions that, in the administration's eyes, are where the real money is. This is one of the paradoxes of our practice. We work hard to keep patients out of the hospital but exist because of the patients who get admitted.

## Shifting Boundaries in the Home Care Setting

As invited guests in patients' homes, we are always aware that traditional boundaries have subtly shifted. Sometimes we are treated like trusted family members, which can be helpful when reassuring patients and caregivers that a new diagnosis will be treatable or that a certain lump is really nothing to be concerned about. But sometimes the familiarity fostered by home visits can be frustrating: medical providers are generally accustomed to having a certain degree of authority, which can seem diluted in this less formal setting. Despite these ups and downs, the process of developing mutual respect and time spent learning about each other help patients and caregivers build strong and productive clinical relationships with their medical providers.

For our physicians and nurse practitioners, going into the home permits a greater understanding of medical and non-medical issues. Poverty, abuse, neglect, safety, isolation—the "home biopsy" that is possible with firsthand observation reveals much that is otherwise inaccessible in even the most directed clinical interview. The contents or emptiness of a refrigerator, a stack of unopened bills, a family member's desperate sign on the door reminding the patient not to go outside—these things can tell volumes about how well a patient is living.

A home visit makes it impossible to ignore the plight of the patient living in a sixth-floor walk-up, or unable to enter the bathroom in her wheelchair. Half-eaten food and uncollected garbage may flag the need for more support services. The state of medical equipment may reveal how appropriate it is: has the bedside commode, for example, been turned into a nightstand because the patient is now able to walk to the bathroom again, or because he was unable to use it without a home attendant to help him empty and clean it? Like detectives, we strive to interpret the details that reveal a diagnosis and help in developing a treatment plan.

## Vulnerable Patients, Vulnerable Caregivers

Home visiting reminds us how deceptive first impressions can be. Marino Roman's referral by a nursing agency initially seemed unnecessary: a confident female voice announced through the downstairs intercom, "I'm his daughter, things are just fine. I'm on sabbatical from work and—" when a small, dry voice in the background called out, "She's my wife—please come up! Don't listen to her! She's my wife!" After the building superintendent let us in with the dry comment, "Oh yeah, 4E; somebody needs to do something about them," we found Mr. Roman standing in the doorway, a tiny, disheveled man bent almost halfway over, held up by a wobbling cane. His clothes smelled strongly of urine. Behind him was a woman in similarly shabby dress, suspiciously glaring at us. Asking permission to come in, we entered. Mr. Roman stated, "She has memory problems. I don't know what to do."

The story unfolded. Mr. Roman suffered from Parkinson's disease, hypothyroidism, and prostate disease, while his wife, Sunny, had regressed into a paranoid state as her dementia worsened. She was fixated on the idea that she was forty years younger and taking a break from her work, probably identifying with their daughter, who died in a car accident years earlier. While the Romans were in sporadic telephone contact with their son-in-law and grandchildren, who lived in California, no one knew how bad things were.

The apartment had become severely dilapidated, and the Romans were struggling to care for each other. Mr. Roman had great difficulty getting to the bathroom. Neither could manage to cook; instead they ordered in, which they could not afford. Sometimes Mrs. Roman would leave the apartment, because Mr. Roman did not have the physical strength to stop her, and he was terrified that she might not find her way back.

A few coordinated telephone calls organized a home health aide, a visiting nurse, and physical therapy for Mr. Roman. The son-in-law, now aware of the desperate situation, arranged for new beds to replace the Romans' old broken and soiled ones. Cultivating Mrs. Roman's trust so that she would allow a physical examination and basic blood tests was more difficult. After several visits, she relented, and tests revealed severe hypothyroidism, which was worsening her dementia; with the initiation of new medication, she became less labile and moody. Mr. Roman also benefited from adjustments to his medication regimen. He was quietly bemused as he said in the same small, dry voice that had recently called out for help, "I'm clean and I have clean clothes. I am not worried now about us being so alone."

## What Caregivers Want: Basic and Humane Care

In the vast majority of cases, we find, caregivers aren't asking for miracles. They simply want basic and humane care for their loved ones. They need help in solving problems. They need someone other than themselves to be responsible for communicating medical information. They need us to keep their own needs and preferences in mind.

Charles Eisen, an 80-year-old man who lived with Katherine, his wife of 55 years, was referred to the program because of his refusal to leave their home to see a doctor. In fact, he refused to leave the apartment for any reason, even though he was clearly losing weight, felt weak, barely ate, and spent almost all of his time in bed. His medical history included a diagnosis of small-cell lung cancer, which had been surgically treated one year earlier, a previous heart attack, and emphysema. Mrs. Eisen worried and was keenly frustrated because she could not figure out how to help him. If she left his bedside for a minute he would grow frantic and call out for her—twice he fell while trying to get out of bed when she had left the room. She called his various specialists, scheduling appointments that her husband would not keep. The doctors, in turn, were reluctant to treat Mr. Eisen over the telephone or renew medications without first seeing him. Mrs. Eisen requested copies of his medical records from previous hospitalizations, which she took to friends and friends of friends who were doctors, but they too were reluctant and unsure about how to become involved. They urged her to bring him to the hospital. It was one of these friends who recommended our home-visiting program.

At our initial meeting, Katherine Eisen was apologetic and wary, yet eager to get something done. "He already has several top specialists. He's known them for years." Charles Eisen lay in bed, each intake of breath a visible struggle of mind over matter. Eyeing me with skepticism, he clearly thought I had come to spirit him away to the hospital against his will. Instead, as I sat at his bedside after the physical exam, medical history, and evaluation of his symptoms, we explored several scenarios. We bargained over each possible option—blood tests, a hospital bed, oxygen, medication changes, hospitalization, and evaluations by specialists. His wife implored him to allow "everything" to be done to find out what was happening to his body.

Eventually we reached a compromise that was acceptable to him: just blood tests and a change of medications to treat severe breathlessness and pain. Mrs. Eisen was upset, but she acquiesced to what her husband wanted. She called the Visiting Doctors office frequently for advice on managing his constipation, lack of appetite, and cough. She met with the social worker to cope with her feelings of anger at her husband for what she thought were bad decisions, and at herself for becoming angry with him. She was troubled by her feelings of helplessness. Six months later, Mr. Eisen finally agreed to a radiology appointment, and a chest x-ray confirmed a recurrence of his lung cancer.

It was revealing to see how, after months of arguing over the utility of CT scans, blood tests, and the best that the academic medical center's brain trust could offer, he wanted only to be pain free, at home with his wife. Once he knew the bad news, his primary concern was for her. At the next home visit, she had fallen asleep in a chair next to his bed. "I'm more worried about Katherine than myself," he whispered. We were struck by how he wanted our help with this deeply personal matter of preparing her for his death. Considering how we had bartered and negotiated over the last year, we had thought that the home visits had not mattered to him beyond the practical aspects of pain and symptom management.

When Mrs. Eisen woke up, we all discussed her husband's advance directive and his decision to die at home with only comfort care. Both agreed to accept additional hospice services that they had previously refused. At a home visit two weeks later, Mr. Eisen was at peace, comfortable, and barely conscious. We talked with a calm but tearful Mrs. Eisen about what to expect as he drew closer to death. Half an hour after we left she called to tell us he had died. She said she would never have been able to make it through the past year without going crazy if it had not been for the team's consistent emotional support, patience, and willingness to meet her and her husband on their own terms.

## Multidisciplinary Teamwork, Multiple Viewpoints

At best, the discussion of "how much do you understand about your illness," "what is the most important thing to you now," and "what would you want me to do or not do as you get sicker and face death" evolves over months to years of respectful partnership. This works well when patients are referred to our program at an early enough stage to permit a natural progression of the conversation. Unfortunately, we do not always have the

luxury of time in which to help caregivers and patients make critical decisions. Many patients are referred to our program only months from death.
Whether early or late in the process, we rely on frequent interdisciplinary
team meetings and early referrals to our social worker when patients and
families are overwhelmed.

As a team, we work hard to foster an environment in which every
member is able to act as a patient advocate. Administrative assistants
who answer the phones are often the first to detect increased levels of
depression, frustration, or anxiety in a patient or caregiver. Our Spanish-
language translator does much more than simply convert words from one
language into another. She is both a cultural liaison and a very careful ob-
server—frequently picking up clues to complex family relationships that
would otherwise be overlooked. The benefits of this approach are self-evi-
dent, though it is certainly not without conflict. Multiple voices can mean
multiple differing viewpoints.

Different viewpoints among team members are particularly common
in the care of what are euphemistically called "difficult" patients. These
are patients who, for one reason or another, thwart every effort to help
them. They rarely take their medications, refuse to accept desperately
needed home care services (such as wound care for a festering ulcer), and
are verbally abusive to our staff. We meet them because their previous
doctors have given up on them, or they refuse to leave their apartments
to seek help. We know, almost from the first visit, that our ability to have a
positive impact on their lives will be quite limited. Yet we suspect that we
are their last chance for help. So we struggle to maintain contact.

Team conflict generally arises when one member, usually the patient's
doctor or nurse practitioner, can't take it anymore. He or she becomes
convinced that we are doing no good in staying involved in the patient's
care, and that it would be better for all concerned to end the relationship.
Rarely is there an immediate consensus that this should be the case. Other
team members might point out that we are providing a valuable service
in supporting the patient's informal caregivers. Still others might point
out that, in their own interactions with the patient, he or she is becoming more receptive to participating in the care plan. Our interdisciplinary
meetings provide an important forum where all of these viewpoints can
be expressed. In the end, we are usually able to gain further insight into
what might best help the patient and the caregivers.

## Helping Caregivers Set Limits

We have also come to recognize that not every patient should remain at home, even when all parties wish it. Anna Guyton, for example, was diagnosed with a brain tumor three years ago. She suffers from recurrent seizures and has become severely debilitated. Despite both chemotherapy and radiation, there has been little change in the tumor. She is blind, paralyzed on her left side, and has difficulty swallowing. It can take an hour to feed her a cup of oatmeal. Anna's granddaughter, Carmen Mitchell, recently moved Anna into her own home to care for her. Carmen is a single parent to young twin sons, Clay and Andy. Andy attends a special school for learning-disabled children and takes several medications for his hyperactivity syndrome.

Stretched between her job, Andy's special needs, Clay's feeling left out, and her grandmother's care, Carmen was greatly relieved when she was first referred, by a relative, to the Visiting Doctors program. She did not have to coordinate doctor's visits and she knew that, if she picked up the phone with a question, she would get a prompt answer. Newly prescribed medications also helped ease Anna's symptoms. Home health aides tended to Anna's physical care during the day. The situation began to deteriorate, however, when Anna's seizures became more frequent, terrifying the entire family. Additionally, Anna required several trips to the emergency room for intravenous medications to control the intractable convulsions. After one such episode, when Anna developed pneumonia, the interdisciplinary team met with Carmen in the hospital to discuss what to do.

Torn between her promise to do the best for her grandmother and the work of raising two boys on her own, Carmen faced a difficult choice. It was clear that she had made a Herculean effort to keep Anna with the family, but that Anna's medical needs had reached a level of intensity that was logistically impossible to handle at home. Together, the family and Visiting Doctors team explored the options. Ultimately, they decided that an inpatient hospice was the best place for Anna to receive the specialized care she needed while allowing Carmen and her boys to focus on being loving family members, rather than having to be managers of the treatment regimen. In this case, the family needed help in setting appropriate limits; for the Visiting Doctors, the challenge was to avoid fostering unrealistic expectations, while remaining steadfast in our commitment to the patient and the family, and being as creative as possible in exploring options and alternatives.

## The Value of Supportive Relationships

Caregivers sometimes have unmet emotional needs that medical providers may be unaware of—or unequipped to address. In such cases, the value of an interdisciplinary approach to care cannot be overstated. Tracy Maurice's husband, Walter, had Parkinson's disease. When Walter's medical provider became aware of the great strain Mrs. Maurice was experiencing, she referred her to our program's social worker for supportive counseling. The social worker began meeting with Mrs. Maurice in her home every other week.

Mrs. Maurice was facing great challenges caring for her husband at home. Mr. Maurice was no longer the partner he had once been. Every day his wife watched the signs of his progressive deterioration. Yet she rarely had the time to mourn this incredible loss, because she was occupied with the tasks of his care. Although she had a personal care aide for him, she believed that nobody else would take as good care of Walter as she would. She was exhausted by the amount of attention she gave him and felt guilty about taking time for herself. She missed "the old Walter" terribly. And her grief was more pronounced when she was with him because, although he was present in body, his mental state was profoundly diminished.

Caregivers who choose to keep their family members at home are asked to become experts in areas with which they may have no experience or level of comfort. Mrs. Maurice took on all sorts of new responsibilities in caring for her husband. She became case manager—coordinating all the providers who came into the home, including doctors, nurses, physical therapists, and aides. She was asked to observe and report on her husband's symptoms, appetite, reaction to medications, bodily functions, and behaviors, as if she were a clinician herself. She had to become an advocate—searching out services and benefits while learning to understand the complexities of health care coverage. And she had to assume responsibility for all household finances.

Mrs. Maurice was in her eighties. She had never been a supervisor before, certainly not of home attendants, who need to be trained to meet the specific needs of each patient. She had to orient them to her house and adjust to having new people in her kitchen, bedroom, and living room all day long. This loss of privacy and dignity was particularly uncomfortable for her. She remarked on how difficult it was for her to give up her kitchen, as the home attendant slowly reorganized it for her own work style. These combined challenges strained Mrs. Maurice's own health.

With the social worker, Mrs. Maurice explored how she might begin taking time out for herself through socializing and exercise. These were difficult steps. Anything that involved making a commitment to leave the house became stressful because she never knew what would come up while she was out. Because of Mrs. Maurice's reluctance to leave the home for her own appointments, the in-home social work visits proved to be quite valuable to her. She benefited a great deal from the opportunity to unload, to cry, and to be heard—things that she had not been able to do prior to these visits.

For Mrs. Maurice, alleviation of her stress and anxiety came through a process of establishing a supportive relationship. In the past, she had endured a string of strained relationships with medical providers of whom she felt distrustful, and who in turn perceived her as demanding and meddlesome. The social worker also helped Mr. Maurice's doctor appreciate Mrs. Maurice's fear and need to be overly responsible for the care of her husband. This was an important step in fostering the development of a strong collaborative bond between the doctor and Mrs. Maurice. The collaborative model of the Visiting Doctors program nurtured a sense of mutual respect, and established a support system that allowed the Maurices to feel less alone.

## Making a Difference

There are many other homebound patients, and caregivers, like the Maurices, Mrs. Brown, the Romans, and the Eisens, in Manhattan and all across the United States. Each referral is more than "end-stage dementia," "metastatic colon cancer," or "chronic non-compliance." Sitting down with people in their own homes has given us all a greater insight into what it is like to be sick or old, very poor or alone. We have also seen the impact of thoughtful, dedicated caregiving and the difference it can make, no matter what the medical diagnosis or home setting.

The services we provide are only a drop in the proverbial bucket compared to the vast depth of need that patients and families encounter daily. But for our team, the myriad challenges of providing intensive home care to the old, the disabled, and the most marginalized members of society make this the toughest job we have ever faced. It is one that we truly love.

We are constantly reminded of that through encounters with patients like the 92-year-old woman we had been seeing for primary care for three years. As we entered her apartment one day, where she reclined in her hospital bed, beaming, she turned to her new home health aide and, referring to one of our practitioners, declared loudly: "She's not only my doctor, she's also my friend."

# 18 Windows to the Heart: A Family-Centered Hospital Unit for Dementia Patients

*Jeffrey N. Nichols*

Hospitalization is a stressful experience for both patients and family caregivers. That stress is magnified when the patient has cognitive impairments and can neither fully understand what is happening nor communicate fears and concerns. The literature about patients with dementia, primarily with Alzheimer's disease, clearly documents significant functional declines associated with acute hospital care (Mace and Rabins 1999; Sager and Rudberg 1998).

The result, for family caregivers, is a doubly increased burden when their relative is discharged from the hospital: the added level of care needed for the dependent family member, and the further disruption of their own lives. Yet because this phenomenon has largely been assumed to be an inevitable part of dementia, little has been done in response. This chapter describes an attempt to challenge the received wisdom by creating a new culture of care in a hospital unit, in which family caregivers provide an integral part of quality care and in so doing reduce functional decline.

In 1999 Cabrini Medical Center, in New York City, received a six-month planning grant of $20,000 from the United Hospital Fund's Family Caregiving Grant Initiative to assess the needs of family caregivers of our patients (Levine 2003). Because of its location in Lower Manhattan, the 500-bed hospital and its affiliated nursing home serve an ethnically diverse population, including many non-English-speaking people of Latino and Asian origin. A high proportion of patients are elderly, including many with dementia. Although we had no reliable statistics on the exact proportion of patients in our acute care hospital with dementia, we were fairly sure there were a significant number. Most hospitals do not do good screening for dementia. Moreover, hospital data systems do not capture this information because dementia is not usually the primary diagnosis, and primary diagnoses drive hospital reimbursement. Since approximately 5 percent of community-dwelling seniors and 70 percent of nursing home residents have dementia, we simply assumed that a large number of elderly patients admitted to the hospital have dementia as a significant secondary diagnosis.

### Defining the Problem

To start the planning process, we convened focus groups of family caregivers whose relatives, all with dementia, had recently been hospitalized at Cabrini. The focus groups were run by professional coordinators. We expected family caregivers to tell us that they needed support groups, or more flexible visiting hours, or perhaps better information about the disease and better referrals for follow-up after discharge. We did hear those things.

But even more loudly and clearly, caregivers said that the hospital experience itself was *not* a good one for the patient, or for themselves. They told us that they felt ignored when they came to the hospital, and that although they knew crucial things about what their relative needed, no one seemed interested. They told us that we were often insensitive to the emotional stress that they were undergoing. And they said that what they really would like above all is better care for patients.

The family caregivers were polite but direct. Cabrini Medical Center was no worse than other hospitals, they said. Many of their family members had been patients at other nearby hospitals as well, and *every* hospital was bad in this respect. (We are located in an area of New York known in the community as "Bedpan Alley" because there are literally thousands of hospital beds within a few square miles. Sometimes it is a matter of chance where an ambulance takes a patient.) We concluded that we were dealing with an aspect of generally accepted institutional culture that has profound, long-lasting, detrimental effects on vulnerable patients.

From their perspectives these family caregivers reinforced what we knew from the literature. They brought to the hospital patients who were moderately functional but had some acute medical problem like pneumonia. When the patients were discharged, the acute problem was resolved but baseline functional status was dramatically worse. What is more, in the course of the hospitalization both family caregivers and the persons they care for were subjected to painful and humiliating experiences. Family caregivers of nursing home residents echoed those observations about the effects of hospitalization.

## Levers for Change

Somewhat surprisingly, and for a number of reasons, the hospital leadership was willing to listen to this disconcerting message. First, the United Hospital Fund's Family Caregiving Initiative stimulated the hospital to focus on family caregivers' needs. When foundations fund initiatives, they are able to bring attention to previously unaddressed issues.

A second very influential factor was the personal experiences of individuals in senior hospital administration who were caregivers themselves and whose relatives had been hospitalized. The stories from the focus groups had a special resonance for them. This is not so surprising. Large numbers of Americans serve as family caregivers and many of them are middle-aged. It naturally follows that at practically every hospital there are senior staff who are also family caregivers. We were fortunate that many of the people we invited to help us think about the project had these experiences, and subsequently supported the project.

Third, our facility is sponsored by a religious order, the Missionary Sisters of the Sacred Heart of Jesus, familiarly known as the Cabrini Sisters. Our hospital takes seriously its mission to provide family-centered care, and to translate into practice our dedication to a purpose higher than simply moving patients in and out of the hospital. The name we gave to the unit we would develop—Windows to the Heart—reflects both its goal and Cabrinian sponsorship.

## A New Culture of Care

To follow up on the results of the focus groups, we brought together a group of senior administrators from both Cabrini Medical Center and Cabrini Center for Nursing and Rehabilitation, its affiliated nursing home, and said, "If this is what's broken, how do we go about fixing it?" The more we talked, the clearer it became that we could not accomplish our goal in a piecemeal fashion—tweak this, tweak that, and expect significant improvement. We realized that we needed to change the whole culture of care—the way we interacted with families and the way we took care of patients suffering from dementia. This change would affect staff job descriptions, the nature of their work, and what was considered important and not important.

The new culture of care had to both respect and involve family caregivers. We could no longer see family caregivers and their needs as just another problem to deal with, one that staff might have some time to address on a "good" day. In the current hospital environment, "good" days are rare. We felt that care would not change if we just patched a little extra time on top of a bad situation, especially if that extra time was grant funded.

Indeed, the project had to be something that would make other people realize, "We can do that." We wanted to be able to show that units like this could be created with only a modest financial outlay. For the hospital, that meant a capital contribution of approximately $90,000 for construction. The bulk of development costs were covered by a two-year United Hospital Fund implementation grant of $175,000. With that we were able to move ahead to create Windows to the Heart as an eight-bed, family-centered acute care hospital unit for patients with dementia. (A similar unit was also created at the Cabrini Center for Nursing and Rehabilitation. Because the process and problems were rather different, they will be discussed separately in this chapter.) Later, in 2001, an additional grant of $75,000 allowed us to enhance the program and publicize our experience.

Coincidentally, while we were planning our approach, the National Alzheimer's Association held a retreat in which they, too, concluded that hospital care of Alzheimer's patients was a major unaddressed area. They envisioned funding a hospital-based project to improve some aspects of care. Then they heard through their New York chapter, our community-based partner in this effort, that we were already embarking upon such a project. When the Alzheimer's Association representatives came to visit, they discovered that we were trying to address the issues they had identified. We were ambitiously attempting to fix all the problems at the same time! But perhaps that was the only way it actually could be done: I would argue that revolution, not evolution, is the only route that leads to the goal of profound cultural change.

## Barriers to Change and Strategies for Overcoming Them

Beyond questions of ongoing funding, perhaps the greatest barrier we anticipated was the prevailing belief that change was impossible. We knew we would need unconditional support from senior hospital administration because what we were proposing cut across many different boundaries and had the potential to upset so many different staff members. We wanted to make sure that everyone whose department was going to be affected blessed the project in advance. We did not want to find out we could not implement the project because it was being secretly undermined by people with different priorities or needs.

We tried very consciously to involve everybody in the senior administration relatively early, to let each one know what we were doing. We said openly, "These are things that are going to be different, is that all right with you? Is that going to be a problem? Tell us what the problem is in advance." We tried to prepare for a wide variety of contingencies, and were ready for administrative opposition ranging from open hostility to ostensible friendliness that masked foot-dragging obstructionism.

In any large bureaucracy, people who have not been consulted are inevitably going to have concerns. Very often, however, if they are involved in solving or even framing the problem they are much more invested in the success of the project. And when you are genuinely inclusive and respectful of people's legitimate concerns, they will usually find ways to work with you and not against you.

The process of winning support occurred at several levels. We engaged Dr. Jacalyn Sherriton, president of Health Management Consultants, Inc., to facilitate a series of meetings. Those with senior management helped locate the unit within the hospital's administrative structure and set allowable parameters for change. Meetings with middle managers allowed them to remain informed and to formally assent to proposed changes. And those with project staff were helpful in team building. Dr. Judah Ronch, a clinical psychologist, conducted another series of meetings with the professionals and nonprofessionals from all three weekday and weekend shifts who would comprise the unit staff, to rethink how the unit would function within the new cultural paradigm. Unit staff accepted the new model enthusiastically, possibly because this person- and family-centered care was completely consistent with their professional training, their own personal experiences and values, and the hospital's mission.

We involved the directors of medicine and nursing, the heads of food service, pharmacy, housekeeping, security, social work, discharge planning, chaplaincy, senior nursing administration, and senior medical personnel. If we planned to change visiting hours, we knew it would be important to involve the admitting office and security. We tried to include everyone who might be affected by our efforts to change the culture of care.

Initially, there was considerable concern. The human-resources administrators, for example, were worried that union personnel might object to anything that appeared to change job descriptions and reporting channels. We were careful about how we went about making changes, and it turned out to *not* really be an issue. In the end, hospital staff identified fewer potential problems than we anticipated: people were more flexible, more understanding of what the needs were going to be, than we had originally expected.

We knew, for example, that we were going to need extra time from the social service staff. Rather than scheduling the extra meetings and then hearing from the director of social service that "my staff doesn't have time to come to all these meetings; we've got other things to do," we went to her first and said, "How much time can you commit for your staff to attend the extra meetings that we know are going to be necessary? We are not going to schedule more time than you think they can reasonably provide." With this approach she actually offered a larger number of hours than we would have asked for. At that point, it became an accepted part of the social work staff's responsibility to attend these meetings.

Remarkably, this process proceeded throughout a period of extreme financial instability in the hospital. As the administration cut staff, various team members lost their positions and were either not replaced at all or were replaced by others who had not participated in the program design. During the grant period the hospital had three chief executive officers, four chief operating officers, four directors of nursing, three chief medical officers, and a parade of vice-presidents and consultants with enough tables of organization to deplete a modest-sized forest. Despite this constant disruption—and the turmoil in Lower Manhattan created by the World Trade Center attack—Windows to the Heart managed to thrive. It has been included in every strategic plan from administration, consultants, and the board of trustees.

## Designing a New Acute Care Unit

In designing the physical layout of our eight-bed unit, we consulted with Lorraine Hiatt, an expert in creating nursing home dementia units and adult daycare programs. She advised us on how, working within a limited budget, we could make the space responsive to the needs of people with dementia.

The available space was part of a very large hospital unit that included a series of two-bed rooms and a corner four-bed room. By removing the beds and wall equipment from the corner room, we created a caregiver and patient lounge. We added couches and a chair that turns into a daybed, built a wheelchair-accessible bathroom and a family caregiver bathroom, and installed shelves to hold educational materials. The room has dining tables, because dementia patients tend to eat better in a social setting. The hallway has grab bars. With prior approval from Infection Control we carpeted the lounge and the hallways. The two-bed rooms remained nearly as they had been. We repainted them in neutral colors and upgraded the lighting, because shadows and odd lighting tend to induce paranoia and fear in patients suffering from dementia.

One basic principle of Alzheimer's design is to make things *look* as much like what they're supposed to be as possible. Outlining a door in color helps people recognize that it is, in fact, a door. Things that you *don't* want people to notice should be the same color as the background. The stairwell that goes down to the street, for example, is painted in the same color as its background wall. Since some of our patients tend to wander, the general color scheme and layout of the unit encourage people to move in the direction of the caregiver room, which is where we want people to congregate.

We were very aware that repetitive, loud, hostile sounds are confusing and disruptive for patients. Therefore we took the extraordinary step of removing the telephones and TV sets from the patient rooms. There is a TV in the lounge, where we can control the channel and the volume. Staff bring a portable phone when a patient has a call. As a result the unit is extraordinarily quiet. Some family members complained about the loss of television, but not because they or the patient missed a program. The problem was that paid caregivers who stayed with the patient during the day wanted to watch television, and families were afraid of losing their valued workers. These caregivers are now encouraged to watch television in the family caregiver room when patients are otherwise occupied.

There is no traffic through the unit because it is located on the far corner of the floor. The only reason to come to the unit is because you want to be there. No one wanders through with squeaky carts. No one yells down the corridor, "Get seventeen out of bed to go down for a CAT scan." There is no distracting overhead paging, so the only sounds patients hear are sounds that are *intended*. In addition, we try as much as possible to bring patients to the dayroom where they can interact with other patients and their families in a somewhat more spacious, homelike setting.

We've also been able to tailor some aspects of hospital routine to patient and caregiver needs. Early on, in our planning meetings with unit staff, we asked every member of the team to think, both creatively and concretely, about how their jobs would be different if they were supported in responding to those needs. We considered many of the different tasks involved in daily care. Many of our patients need assistance with eating, for example—being fed, reminded to eat, or cued. This takes a long time. Our dietician arranged to have our unit get its food first and have its trays picked up last, giving us about an extra half-hour. That logistical change allows us additional time to feed our patients, while accommodating the reality of limited staff at mealtimes.

## Staffing and Cost

From the beginning, we built an interdisciplinary team that looks at the patient and the caregiver as a unit, works with them, and responds to the patient's actions as meaningful behavior that needs to be understood. But it was also our intention that, with one exception, there would be no difference in staffing numbers between this and any other unit in the hospital. Part of the reason was practical; there is no point in setting up a unit that requires special funding only to see it disappear after the grant money is gone. Our plan had to be self-sustaining. Our staff is made up primarily of in-house employees reassigned from other units because they choose to participate in this form of care.

The one difference in staffing between our unit and others in the hospital is that a pastoral care worker is assigned almost exclusively to us. She is a bilingual Latin American and has a lot of interaction with Spanish-speaking patients and caregivers and Catholics from other ethnic groups. This is clearly a staffing decision specific to Cabrini.

The grant covered one additional pastoral care position and four consultants—the three previously named, and a research consultant who devised and implemented satisfaction studies. The only other monies from the grant that went toward staff costs, even during the training phase, were for overtime, when we brought in staff from the other shifts so we could gather everybody at the same time for planning and training sessions. These "retreats" were held in the cafeteria.

Cabrini Medical Center is a voluntary hospital, and most patients have private attending physicians. Any attending physician in the Department of Medicine can admit a patient to this unit. Since Windows to the Heart has only eight beds, it does not have its own discrete house staff; we have the same interns and residents as all other units in the hospital.

The geriatricians who provide teaching rounds try to reinforce the two key messages of the unit—that the behavior of patients with dementia is meaningful and that family caregivers can help us understand what those meanings might be. In fact, house staff generally recognize that the care in our unit is different, and that they are expected to behave differently and do different things. They observe that when patients in Beds 6 through 22 get agitated, they can order restraints. But if patients in Beds 23 through 30 become agitated, the standard of care is to go see them and find out why. Still, because of rotating coverage, not every intern or resident has necessarily been educated about the unit and our approach to patient care; in those cases, we find, nurses often provide guidance and advice.

Our unit also has essentially the same nurse staffing as every general medical floor in the hospital. One of the reasons we chose to have eight beds on the unit was that eight beds is the standard assignment for one registered nurse on the day shift. In general, seven of those beds are occupied at any given time.

Where Windows to the Heart staffing differs from other units is in families being able to readily identify the staff involved in a patient's care. Family members had told us that one really difficult thing about the hospital was that they could never figure out who was taking care of their loved one. On most units, assignment sheets are not posted, nobody knows other people's names, and nametags are hard to read. Family members would often spend long periods of time wandering through the floor trying to find somebody who knew whether their father did or did not have breakfast that morning, or whether Mom went for a particular test—and if so whether it was completed, or canceled because she was too upset.

In Windows to the Heart, if a family member walks onto the unit and sees a member of the staff, that staff member is by definition taking care of his or her loved one. The only dietician who comes onto the unit is our dietician. The only social worker present is our unit's social worker. One of the things that the team decided in the course of the planning was that our slogan would be "You can ask anybody because we're all involved in care."

At worst, if a family member asks someone on staff a question and that person does not know the answer, he or she will know who *does* have the answer and can direct the family member appropriately. That has been a major positive aspect of the unit. Staff are empowered to have much more meaningful interaction with family caregivers, and caregivers are spared the demoralizing runaround that is a distressingly familiar feature of traditional institutional care.

## Importance of a Family-Centered Focus

We spent relatively little time actually training people about the disease aspects of dementia. In fact, over the course of almost a year of weekly hour-long meetings, we devoted only two hours to Alzheimer's disease per se. We concluded that most staff don't need to know more of the molecular biology of senile plaques and neurofibrillary tangles to be better at their jobs. What they *do* need is the ability to look at a patient suffering from dementia and respond to him or her as an individual, and to work with a caregiver and understand the importance of what he or she is saying.

One of the reasons taking care of dementia patients in the hospital is so difficult is that they cannot tell us a huge number of things about their daily care—and we send away the person who can, the family caregiver! In fact, caregivers know how their relatives "normally" act, and how to interpret what their nonverbal behavior usually means. If a patient starts rubbing his stomach or pounding the table, it may mean "I need to go to the bathroom," or "I'm bored, I want something to do," or "I'm in pain," or "I'm only comfortable if I have a certain thing around." Before hospitalization, someone was feeding, dressing, and bathing this person every day, and in most cases responding to his or her needs remarkably well. In most hospitals, however, professionals completely ignore caregivers' vast experience and sweep them aside, not realizing that their knowledge is essential if we are to provide the best quality care.

The first question nurses now ask when a patient comes to the unit is, "Who is the caregiver?" We want to find out who knows what this person could do before so that we have some idea of what function it is we are supposed to be preserving. What is it reasonable to expect this patient to be able to do? If we have a problem, whom should we call to get more information? These opening questions represent a completely new approach. Traditionally, nurses might only ask the family member, "Do you have the list of medications?"

In addition, when staff members get the patient's history from caregivers, they ask questions that show they understand dementia and its effects. Staff members are familiar with the kinds of things that people with dementia usually do at home—wandering perhaps, or calling out at night—so they will not just ask about problems or dismiss behavior as bizarre, but will also elicit solutions that have worked at home, and suggestions about what should be done if a problem occurs in the hospital.

Over time, we have tried a number of different ways of getting information from family caregivers. We always ask about feeding, dressing, ambulation, and continence. We try to formulate questions that are more open-ended than directive. Family caregivers do not come in neat packages. Sometimes the caregiver is present at admission and can provide all the information. Sometimes, however, two or three different people may care for an individual, or a family member may supervise a paid caregiver who is the one actually with the patient most of the day.

We keep an independent, relatively informal log on all patients in the unit and share it with the team. This log stays on the unit—it does not become part of the hospital chart—so that if patients are readmitted we do not have to repeat all our questions. The unit has unlimited visiting hours. If family members want to stay over, or feel the patient needs them there, no special permission is required. The family caregiver room has fold-out beds in it for people who want to stay over, and there are fold-out cots available if a caregiver needs to stay in a patient's room. (Because the rooms are two-bedded, however, we encourage caregivers to stay in the lounge instead, unless absolutely necessary, so they don't impinge on the second patient's privacy.) Initially, many family members said they were going to want to stay overnight, but very few have actually done so. Most caregivers felt they needed to stay overnight because, basically, they didn't trust the hospital to take care of their loved one. Once family members recognize that we are both well intentioned and knowledgeable, very few stay overnight.

A remarkable number of relationships have developed among family caregivers. We professional care providers always tend to think it's all about *us*, that family members must want to see *us* for all their information and support needs. In fact, very often one of the benefits for family members of being on the unit is the opportunity to share experiences with other caregivers. Although we have attempted to provide some formal caregiver support, we've found a host of informal interactions going on. For example, when patients need assistance with or reminders about eating, families sometimes will make arrangements with each other—"If you're here this morning to help with my dad, I'll be here this evening to help with your mother."

### Dementia Care in the Nursing Home

Although Cabrini Center for Nursing and Rehabilitation created a 40-bed Dementia Unit at the same time that Windows to the Heart was being developed at the hospital, the process was quite different. First, the nursing home had already made the administrative decision to create a special-ized unit and had begun staff training with the Alzheimer's Association before the initial planning grant was received. Second, numerous models for nursing home dementia units already existed. Indeed, the administra-tion and key staff had visited several of these during the planning phase. Based in part on other facilities' experiences, the administrators had al-ready committed funds for renovations to create a space and support an additional staff person for the proposed dementia activities program.

Additionally, both the nature of long-term care and the nursing home regulatory environment profoundly affect interactions between profes-sional and family caregivers. Obviously, when a resident stays on a floor for months to years, families are readily able to identify staff, learn in-stitutional schedules, and so on. Family participation in nursing home care planning is actually required by federal statute, as is notification of changes in status and family participation in many key decisions, such as the use of physical restraints.

One issue that did arise for the dementia unit related to admissions. The question was not one of identifying residents with dementia, since assessment of cognitive status was already part of the home's routine, but rather *which* of the home's demented residents would most benefit from transfer to a specialized unit.

## Challenges Ahead: Continuity of Care and Appropriate Referral

In the hospital, ensuring continuity of care across units and appropriate referral to Windows to the Heart from the Emergency Department in par-ticular remain unresolved problems. Sometimes a family member will tell other hospital personnel, "Dad was on the dementia unit before, and the staff there seemed to know how to deal with his behavior." But there is no formal mechanism to ensure that patients with dementia will reach us.

We had originally counted on involving the Emergency Department in our planning because we knew, and families have frequently confirmed, that emergency care for patients with dementia is a problem area. Unfor-tunately, during the entire planning period the Emergency Department was administratively short-staffed, with frequent personnel changes, so that no one was able to attend our meetings. Ultimately, their not being involved in the planning process hurt us in a variety of ways.

We have still not been able to establish really effective communica-tions with the Emergency Department. Staff there remain inconsistent in their ability to identify patients appropriate for the unit, in their level of comfort working with caregivers, and in their speed in processing dementia patients through their department. Since dementia is not usually a patient's primary diagnosis, clinicians may not include it as a diagnosis on the chart or may not specify our unit when authorizing or planning an admission. Indeed, they may never even recognize it. The admitting office clerks do not do mental status evaluations, so they cannot identify appropriate patients. The majority of our admissions come through a family member's specifically saying, "I want that unit I read about in the paper." This is an area that we are trying to address in our third-phase "modification" grant.

Alternatively, patients may have been admitted to a different floor until they exhibited "problem" behaviors and were reassigned to us. We are the place in the hospital that *wants* the patient who is wandering or disrupting the sleep of patients on regular medical and surgical floors. A few attending physicians specifically request the unit for their dementia patients, and none have objected to patient placement there. But most attending physicians have had difficulty understanding the unit and its purpose, since specialized units in hospitals, like cardiac care units, usually revolve around the patient's primary diagnosis. Because dementia is so often a co-morbidity, it is very difficult to get these patients into the system appropriately.

## Bringing Best Dementia Care into the Hospital

Windows to the Heart brings into the acute hospital setting much of what has been known for some time about good long-term dementia care. It is hard to look at some of the specific aspects of our new culture of care and see them as so remarkable if you are familiar with what good assisted living programs, good adult daycare programs, good Alzheimer's units and skilled nursing facilities have been doing for years. We certainly did not invent interdisciplinary care. Almost all the behavioral approaches we use have been known to people in other contexts. But insofar as hospitals see themselves at the top of the care system, they have exhibited an institutional arrogance—unprepared or unwilling to listen to what people in rehabilitation settings or long-term care know, and to incorporate that knowledge into the hospital's culture and systems of care.

A major advantage at Cabrini is that we are a hospital connected to a nursing home; I am the chief of geriatrics in the hospital as well as medical director of the nursing home. This dual role means that I am able to go back and forth between the two different worlds and say, "These challenges can be tackled."

One of the things we have struggled against is the notion that there are prefabricated solutions for problems. Instead of coming up with a model for others to replicate, our approach has been a problem-solving one. We never expected that this unit was going to be *the* model that everybody else would use. Rather, we have pragmatically addressed the many challenges to show what *could* be accomplished. Most of what we did we made up along the way. I can imagine this unit looking very different, perhaps being staffed differently, and functioning differently. As proud as I am of everything we have done, I certainly recognize the limitations. While we have anecdotal evidence that patients leave our unit less debilitated, and their caregivers more satisfied, than the norm, we have yet to gather rigorous data to that effect. But it is the process, and not necessarily the model, that is really important.

## Acknowledgments

Some of the material in this chapter appeared in different form in Nichols JN and KS Heller, 2001, Windows to the Heart: Creating an acute care dementia unit [interview], *Innovations in End-of-Life Care* 3(2). www2.edc. org/lastacts/archives/archivesMarch01/featureinn.asp Accessed July 21, 2004; in *Journal of Palliative Medicine* 5(1) (2002): 181-92; and in Romer AL, KS Heller, DE Weissman, and MZ Solomon, eds., 2002, *Innovations in end-of-life care: Practical strategies and international perspectives*, vol. 3 (Larchmont, NY: Mary Ann Liebert).

## References

Levine C. 2003. *Making room for family caregivers: Seven innovative hospital programs*. New York: United Hospital Fund.

Mace NL and PV Rabins. 1999. *The 36-hour day. A family guide to caring for persons with Alzheimer disease, related dementing illnesses, and memory loss in later life.* 3rd ed. Baltimore: Johns Hopkins University Press.

Sager MA and MA Rudberg. 1998. Functional decline associated with hospitalization for acute illness. *Clinics in Geriatric Medicine* 14(4): 669-79.

# 19     Connecting Caregivers through Technology

*Andrea Y. Hart*

For family caregivers, the technology that has so vastly eased and expanded the scope of communications in recent years is more than just a convenience: Internet and telecommunications forums are virtual lifelines, affording fast access to information and resources, linking caregivers to others in similar situations, and relieving some of the isolation that is endemic to caregiving. Although many family caregivers are older women—not the expected Web-surfing demographic—one study has found older caregivers as likely as their younger counterparts to use the Internet if they have access to it (White and Dorman 2000).

While searching caregiver or health-related Web sites for information is an important part of caregivers' computer use, this chapter focuses primarily on how caregivers are using various interactive technologies to obtain social and emotional support. It begins with a review of the kinds of online and telecommunications resources available and a look at the range of issues covered, as exemplified by a selection of current peer and professional forums. From there, the chapter moves on to the kind of information and support caregivers seek, the advantages and disadvantages of these newer technologies, and caregivers' preferences for receiving support, before concluding with lessons learned from current and former organizers, and recommendations for creating successful interactive caregiver support groups.

## Interactive Formats

Computer- and, to a lesser extent, telephone-based technologies offer a variety of ways to access information and to join virtual communities. These resources may operate synchronously (in real time), permitting simultaneous interaction among participants, or asynchronously, allowing users to participate as their schedules permit (Perron 2002). They may have open memberships or require registration and a password for participation; in the latter type, especially, there is often a professional moderator to facilitate discussions, answer clinical or other enquiries, and/or ensure adherence to group guidelines. Community formats include:

- *Listservs*, e-mail groups for individuals interested in a specific topic or members of a specific organization. These can have open or closed memberships and may be moderated. Individuals subscribe to a listserv via the organizer's Web site; messages are posted to a central address and then forwarded to all members. This asynchronous model allows users to reply to the entire mailing list or direct a more personal response to another member;

- *Newsgroups,* also open to members of the public with an interest in a particular issue. Messages usually relate to news stories, new reports, or other factual information about the selected topic;

- *Chat rooms/chat sessions,* virtual communities that operate in real time. Chat sessions are usually held at a specified time, for several individuals or the entire community, and may be professionally moderated;

- *Bulletin boards,* allowing messages to be posted at users' convenience. Individuals can skim posts, respond to specific messages, or write their own. Some bulletin boards feature an "anger wall" where participants can post "charged" messages. Many have an "Ask the Expert" section where queries can be posted to professionals;

- *Teleconferencing,* updating standard telephone technology to allow multiple parties to converse at the same time. Participants are linked by dialing a toll-free number or are called at the prearranged time by an operator or the sponsor/organizer;

- *Computer-mediated systems*, currently under development. These password-protected networks, using a voice data system or adapted computer device, link caregivers with one another, other family members, health professionals, and information and assistance resources. The various systems may include features such as bulletin boards, decision-support systems, personal mailboxes, and respite components.

## Innovative Programs

Interactive communities may feature general discussions open to anyone interested in the broad issue of caregiving, or may be narrowly focused. The sheer number and variety of caregiver forums is overwhelming: a Web search for "Internet caregiver groups" will turn up thousands of links and references, many of which are duplicates or nonfunctioning sites (COR Health 2001).

Finding the right forum can be a challenge, depending on the commonality the caregiver seeks. By its very nature, for example, Alzheimer's disease is one of the conditions in which considerable attention has been directed to the caregiver (White and Dorman 2000). The Alzheimer's Association sponsors several Web sites that provide disease-related information, caregiver support, and links to other resources. Caregivers of persons with rare, so-called orphan diseases will clearly have fewer choices. Still, many other single-interest organizations have begun to address caregiver needs as well—not only disease-specific groups but also those serving particular classes of caregivers, whether linked by their relationship to care recipients, religious or racial backgrounds, age, or sexual orientation. Even a small sampling of currently functioning programs illustrates the range available (a more extensive list of interactive groups can be found in Chapter 20).

### Professionally Led Groups

- CancerCare, a national organization with headquarters in New York City, provides free counseling, information, referrals, and direct financial assistance to persons with cancer and their families. CancerCare's mission is to educate patients, caregivers, and relatives of cancer patients about the disease and developments in treatment, and to offer support and coping strategies. Its closed bulletin board, with sessions professionally moderated by oncology social workers, first went online in 1997.

- Family Caregiver Alliance (FCA), based in San Francisco, offers a variety of forums for family caregivers, including a general caregiver listserv, and networks for caregivers of persons with brain injury, Huntington's and Parkinson's diseases, multiple sclerosis, and other motor disorders, and for gay, lesbian, bisexual, and transgender caregivers. In 2000, FCA launched Links2Care, an Internet program for caregivers of California residents with dementing illnesses. A computer-mediated system modeled after the CHESS (Comprehensive Health Enhancement Support System) network created at the University of Wisconsin, Madison, Links2Care features a moderated closed listserv, decision-support network, library, database of community resources, and access to experts.

- AlzOnline—a collaboration of the State of Florida Department of Elder Affairs, the University of Florida (UF), and the UF Center on Telehealth and Healthcare Communications—is a professionally facilitated telephone and online intervention for caregivers of persons with progressive dementia. Using "positive caregiving classes," the site delivers educational, informational, and skills support in English and Spanish; a bulletin board is also available.

- New York City's Beth Israel Medical Center Department of Pain Medicine and Palliative Care has operated Net of Care, a network for caregivers of the medically ill, since 2001. Programs include an ongoing telephone-based support group in English and Spanish; a series of one-hour Webcasts, featuring lectures and question-and-answer sessions, designed "to alleviate distress and promote coping skills"; and www.NetofCare.org, an online interactive Web site that features a database of local and national resources, a newsletter, a caregiver distress scale, and other informational and "how-to" materials, such as a caregiver resource guide that can be downloaded and printed.

- DOROT, a multiservice agency in New York City that assists the homebound and homeless elderly, developed Caregivers' Connections in 2001. These interactive teleconferences, led by professional facilitators, offer emotional support to caregivers of the elderly and help them access community resources.

- In Dallas, the North Texas Health Care System/VA Hospital-Dallas has been operating The Conversation Call, a telephone forum created to disseminate information and educational tools on the effects of dementia. For the past two years the moderated forum has focused on delivering information to caregivers in a standardized format.

*Peer-Led Groups*

While many support networks are facilitated by health care or social work professionals, family caregivers themselves are working vigorously as well to help others cope.

- Caregivers in Action, a Baltimore-based support group for caregivers of elderly, disabled, and chronically ill persons, was founded in 1989 by a behavioral scientist with 18 years of caregiving experience. In 2001, Caregivers in Action implemented telephone and Internet support in an effort to reach caregivers who had no access to traditional face-to-face gatherings. Telephone sessions are one-on-one; Internet-based support consists of a weekly chat session and a bulletin board moderated by the founder—experts are periodically invited to join in.

- Empowering Caregivers, an online intervention created by a caregiver, is affiliated with the National Organization for Empowering Caregivers. The Web site offers emotional and spiritual support via a bulletin board, chat room, online newsletter, articles, and other resources.

Sometimes professionally led groups become more caregiver directed over time, or extend beyond the initial boundaries of phone or Internet contact. One study's researchers noted that conversations initially led by facilitators were increasingly directed by group members—who selected topics they felt important and guided the flow of sessions—as they became more comfortable with one another (Stewart et al. 2001). Moreover, weekly calls that had been planned to run 45 minutes averaged 105 minutes, and at the conclusion of the 12-week series caregivers exchanged contact information and planned to meet. In another study of telephone support, as well, group members expressed such a high level of interest in one another that they, too, decided to meet for lunch (Gitlin 2002).

## The Search for Advice and Support

Although the original and still primary purpose of many Internet groups is to provide emotional support and an outlet for caregivers' frustrations, many focus instead on caregivers' need for information and advice, whether on major care decisions that need to be made, or a baffling, still-not-diagnosed condition. These sites enable users to exchange information on possible diagnoses, complementary and alternative treatments, drug therapies, and clinical trials (Klemm, Reppert, and Visich 1998) that may not have been covered or understood during discussions with the health care team. In fact, caregivers are the largest segment of Internet users to conduct searches for treatments and mental health information (Fox and Fallows 2003). Group members also convey information about health professionals, community resources, and material support (Stewart et al. 2001). And participants often pass on their own techniques for providing better patient care. In Dallas, for example, one organizer stated, "The Conversation Call helps caregivers not only learn to talk to one another but also to see each other as resources for learning practical solutions. One person may have perfected a technique for changing a colostomy bag whereas someone else may be more adept at interacting with a demented patient."

Gathering accurate and timely information to help with decision making gives caregivers a sense of empowerment, and makes it easier to advocate on behalf of care recipients, particularly when speaking with health professionals (Stewart et al. 2001). Support groups may also, in themselves, elicit needed attention from the health care team. That happened with the online forums of Boston's Joslin Diabetes Center, created to help both diabetics themselves and family members seeking to learn "how to best support loved ones with the disease." Finding that queries focused mainly on food and diet prompted the Center to establish a new forum, "Eating for Life," specifically focused on nutrition (Disease Management Advisor 2000).

Exchanges of information are often preludes to more personal interactions. Experience with CancerCare's support groups shows caregivers tending to reach out to others for information before they are open to emotional support. But discussions do commonly evolve to a level of intimacy in which spiritual, financial, and sexual issues are discussed, and frustrations with caregiving duties and with the health care infrastructure itself can be vented. Indeed, emotional support remains at the core of many groups and conversations. A recent review of e-mail and bulletin board groups found that nearly two-thirds (61.87 percent) of messages were related to emotions (Perron 2002).

At the same time, general discussions about "normal" life—the weather, family gatherings, the holidays—and moments of shared humor that divert caregivers' attention from their responsibilities (Perron 2002; Pierce, Steiner, and Govoni 2002; White and Dorman 2000) often lead to "virtual" friendships. An elderly caregiver participating in one study of a computer-mediated network cited the "special relationships" cultivated with others in the group (Brennan et al. 1995). Participants in teleconferencing circles, too, note that they have become close personal friends despite never having met. Such strong bonds reflect caregivers' appreciation of being able to communicate with others who have had, and understand, their own or similar experiences (Han and Belcher 2001).

## Pros and Cons of Technology-Mediated Support

Online and telephone support systems encourage individuals to be more forthcoming about their feelings and problems, and help them learn coping strategies and develop networks. In that regard they offer the same benefits as traditional support groups. But technology-based groups have particular advantages of their own—and some unique drawbacks as well.

### Accessibility

Online and telephone networks provide immediate and constant access to caregivers who need to vent, ask a question, or just talk to someone who can empathize (Perron 2002; White and Dorman 2000). Such seven-day, 24-hour accessibility can be crucial since, as the people behind Caregivers in Action understand, professionals are rarely on hand beyond five o'clock. Organizers of that group note that electronic bulletin boards are so effective because caregivers can post messages and receive immediate feedback, rather than contain feelings until they can attend an onsite meeting, when the "heated" moment would have passed without, perhaps, the issue being addressed (White and Dorman 2000). As can many other groups, Caregivers in Action cites occasions when group members were able to respond immediately and provide helpful assistance to a distressed caregiver who found no professional support available.

Equally important, these networks help break down significant barriers posed by disability, geography, and demographics. For the many caregivers who are themselves elderly or disabled, online or telephone communication can mitigate the isolation caused by loss of mobility. For those in rural or suburban areas or without transportation, and those far removed from centers of expertise, networks bridge the distances that would prevent on-site attendance; participants in the Joslin Diabetes Center's forums, for example, came not only from areas surrounding Boston but also from throughout the U.S. and more than 50 other countries

(Disease Management Advisor 2000). Similarly, caregivers of persons with rare conditions can forge a community despite their small numbers.

Still, accessibility is far from universal. Not every household has a computer, and not every caregiver with a computer in the home has the skills to use it. While the cost of personal computers has decreased tremendously, purchasing one and/or paying a monthly fee for Internet access is still not an option for many, especially those caregivers living on fixed incomes and facing major medical and patient-care expenses. For some caregivers, even the cost of telephone service may be prohibitive.

The ease of access that makes the Internet and teleconferencing so attractive can also be problematic, as participants in turn become more accessible to others. Some forum participants find that receiving depressing news, a steady stream of e-mails, and messages unrelated to the topic can adversely affect the online experience (Han and Belcher 2001). So too can group members who engage in "flaming" or the exchange of "emotionally charged" messages (Feldman 2000), and "lurkers," online participants who benefit from the exchange of messages but who themselves do not contribute to the discussion (Perron 2002; Klemm, Reppert, and Visich 1998). Such behavioral issues may be more difficult to tackle than they would be in on-site groups. Identifying "problem" members may be more difficult as well. Online groups are vulnerable to "virtual factitious disorder" or "Munchausen by Internet," in which—just as with Munchausen syndrome's fabrication of illness to attract attention or for other gains—a "forum member" makes up a distressing or disheartening caregiving story that preys on others' sympathies (Feldman 2000). Members reach out with considerable time and support, only to learn eventually that the story is not true, as the individual begins to make contradictory remarks or confuse facts about a disease.

## Anonymity

The anonymity of online and telephone support provides a level of comfort and privacy that does not exist in traditional groups. Even more than in 12-step programs, in which participants do not reveal their full names or other identifiers, membership in an Internet or telephone group affords a sense of confidentiality and safety. This is especially important for caregivers concerned with behavioral health problems such as substance abuse or mental illness, or with other conditions that may either still be stigmatized, such as AIDS, or create problems with insurance for family members, such as the hereditary Huntington's disease. For many caregivers, expressing feelings to "faceless" strangers is far easier than speaking up in on-site meetings or to the health professionals on whom they must rely; without these forums, caregivers who might feel too ashamed or embarrassed to attend traditional meetings, or concerned about value judgments being made about their appearance, dress, or circumstances, would be socially isolated (Stewart et al. 2001).

As with increased access, however, anonymity makes it especially important to scrutinize and weigh the quality of information and Web links offered, and recommendations made, by group participants. One of the drawbacks of anonymity is the cover it provides for persons who join forums to solicit business or sell products or alternative remedies (Disease Management Advisor 2000).

*Convenience*

For caregivers facing the challenges of not enough hours and not enough assistance, access to support directly from home is a huge benefit. With online bulletin boards and listservs available at any time, and no specific amount of time required for participation, many Internet support groups enable caregivers to connect with others at their convenience. Chat rooms, too, allow interaction when formal chats are not scheduled. Although teleconferencing is limited to a specific timeframe, it is made more attractive by requiring no extra expense or complicated set up or other steps to participate. These forums allow live-in caregivers, especially, to "remain at the bedside" without having to deal with finding a substitute caregiver or spend time traveling to and from meeting sites.

Nevertheless, with phone conversations especially, background noise in the caregiver's home can disrupt discussions. And if the care recipient requires close supervision, the caregiver may not be fully attentive to the call or online forum, and may find it difficult to switch from caregiving to "unloading" mode.

*Enhanced Expression*

For many caregivers seeking support, the writing involved in online participation can be very therapeutic (Perron 2002; Pierce, Steiner, and Govoni 2002; White and Dorman 2000). Writers may learn to formulate their thoughts clearly and concisely and to convey their feelings in a creative manner that may be difficult in a traditional support setting (Pierce, Steiner, and Govoni 2002). Whether e-mailing a message to a listserv or posting to a bulletin board, writers can express themselves without inter-ruption; at the same time, they can review and amend messages before sending them, leaving less chance of misinterpretation (Han and Belcher 2001).

Many people find writing difficult and daunting, however, and may therefore be discouraged from taking part in online forums. And with both Internet and teleconferencing groups, nonverbal communication is completely lost, since participants are unable to see each others' facial expressions and body language (Han and Belcher 2001). The "Emoticon" symbols—smiley or sad faces, for example—used in e-mail to convey emotion or comment on written content can be a poor substitute for the nuances of live interaction.

## Assessing User Appeal

Different modalities work for different people, and many organizations offer a number of support groups, using various systems, to accommo-date user preferences. Some caregivers crave the sound of other human voices, while others are happier with exchanges via the keyboard.

Published data and anecdotal reports suggest that individuals are comfortable with technology-mediated support and are willing to sup-plement one type with another. A study of 148 Canadian caregivers of per-sons with dementia looked at whether telephone, newsletter, and com-puter-based support services appealed to respondents, who ranged in age from 21 to 89 (Colantonio, Cohen, and Pon 2001). Only a small fraction al-ready accessed telephone support services, but of the remainder, 66 per-cent expressed interest in professionally led, and 61 percent in peer-led, groups. Moreover, 80 percent of caregivers who would access support via computer indicated they would also participate in a telephone support program staffed by a professional, while 73 percent would do so if there were a peer-led group.

Despite the preference for professional leadership found in the Cana-dian study, one moderator acknowledged that participants in peer-led groups speak more candidly and maintain a higher level of trust and com-fort with one another because of their shared experiences. Hunt (1998) reported that organizers of an online support group from the Cleveland Alzheimer's Association created a forum in which caregivers could access information from experts, but found participants logging on to talk with each other instead.

Yet at least one researcher feels that the efficacy of peer-led groups remains to be adequately demonstrated (Glajchen 2002). And moderators from CancerCare and other organizations note an important benefit of professional involvement: alertness to participants' stress, and the ability to assess caregivers' support systems and needs and to intervene when they encounter a caregiver discussing depression or suicide.

Many forum organizers believe that both peer and professional leadership should be employed. CancerCare, Family Caregiver Alliance, and Alz-Online.net, among other organizations, all clearly recognize the wisdom of "different strokes for different folks." Researchers also support utilizing peer and professional facilitators, because peers "complement" professional intervention (Stewart et al. 2001), and caregivers themselves seem to agree, with many expressing interest in drawing on both formats. In the Canadian study more than three-quarters of the caregivers reported they would access both professional- and peer-led groups rather than one or the other (Colantonio, Cohen, and Pon 2001).

## Creating User-Friendly Services

Organizing and maintaining a technology-aided support group or network can be tremendously rewarding but requires a serious investment of time and energy. Attention to a number of key points maximizes the odds of success.

### A Clear Vision

The most important considerations in planning services are defining and understanding the audience, and ensuring that the service's mission reflects the needs and resources of that target group. Simply having a good idea does not always work, as the Rosalynn Carter Institute, in Americus, Georgia, learned. From 1998 to 2000, the Institute offered Internet support groups to caregivers, but the technology failed to appeal because those in the intended community either did not own computers or were not connected to the Internet (Bauer 2002).

But beyond technical issues, the variety in the caregiving experience suggests that involving caregivers in the design and development of support programs helps organizers better respond to needs. Commonality is, of course, crucial. Caregivers of persons with cognitive dysfunction may require different kinds of support than caregivers of the physically disabled, or of children. And while some caregivers have limited information needs, or want only a periodic outlet for their emotions, others may feel more burdened or more socially isolated and need ongoing or more intense contact—weekly telephone interaction, perhaps, versus checking in occasionally with an Internet bulletin board. Similarly, caregiving may have cycles of varying intensity. CancerCare, for example, has found that many caregivers' responsibilities are reduced, and their need for support decreased, if care recipients' disease goes into remission and they are able to resume many of their previous activities; caregivers may rejoin a group, however, if there is a crisis or recurrence of disease.

### Competent Leadership

Both online and teleconferencing organizers agree that if the group is professionally led, the facilitator should have successful experience working with groups. Some organizers maintain a roster of professionals who can be called on to assist their programs in specific areas of expertise. Professionals responding to messages online, however, must guard against the appearance that they are providing more than just general information. Disclaimers should be posted in e-mail responses and on Web sites, advising participants to consult and follow the advice of their own health care providers (Humphreys, Winzelber, and Klaw 2002). Professionals who provide medical advice should have a backup team of various specialists available to help with responses to complex or discipline-specific questions (Steiner and Pierce 2002).

### Appropriate Access

Controlling the number of participants in interactive-format sessions helps ensure that everyone gets involved in discussions. Some organizers aim for a minimum of five caregivers; others limit participation to a maximum of eight. Most recommend maintaining a waiting list if there are too many potential participants to be placed in a group, or too few—it may be better to hold off on starting a group until there are enough members. Limiting involvement to those living within a specific geographic area, as well, makes it easier to keep track of the resources and services locally available to caregivers.

### Matters of Time

Because caregivers have so much going on in their lives, scheduling problems and no-shows are inevitable. Caregivers may experience sudden crises that prevent them from participating or, at least as likely, may simply forget about a session. To cut down on the latter, some groups find it useful to send out reminders—by e-mail for online sessions or postcard for teleconferences.

### Lay Language

Organizers should recognize that some interested caregivers may not speak (or write) English as their primary language. One of the new computer-mediated systems under development makes it easier to communicate, particularly for non-native speakers, by using a screen phone that transmits voice and text between users (Czaja and Rubert 2002). Automated telephone systems that prompt callers to press specific key pad numbers to indicate yes or no also reduce the likelihood that voice commands will be misinterpreted, and may be helpful not only for those not fluent in English (Mahoney 2000) but also for persons with verbal disabilities. Given the minimal amount of time some caregivers have to participate in online forums, communication should be made easy, with limited typing required and simple language used (Pierce, Steiner, and Govoni 2002).

### The Right Technology

Many organizers believe teleconferencing is an ideal way of extending support because it is a simple modality that does not require caregivers' learning a new skill or acquiring additional equipment. For caregivers it is cost-effective, since most already have a telephone in the home and, in most cases, there is no charge to participate (one organization requests a $10 registration fee but will waive it if a potential group member cannot afford to pay; such fees may help ensure a commitment to participate). Providing toll-free and operator-assisted services can be a costly venture for an organization, however. One study found that teleconferencing charges for groups of four to eleven participants meeting up to two hours a week averaged $300 a session, or roughly $3,000 per group for a ten-week period (Brown et al. 1999). Expenses may be offset through fund-raising, and even by shopping around for teleconferencing services (Stewart et al. 2001). Purchasing a teleconferencing system is an option as well; after recouping the initial outlay it becomes less expensive than contracted services, and ownership allows organizers to maintain total control over calls.

For sponsors of online forums, listservs are perceived to be less complicated than Web-based applications such as bulletin boards and chat rooms, particularly since e-mails are forwarded directly to members' inboxes (COR Health 2001). Web-based applications are not only more prone to technical problems but also require maintenance of their domain names. Losing a domain name most often occurs through "cyber-squatting," when a delayed payment to the Web server allows another party to acquire the site, usually for the value of its name recognition. This means not only having to re-create the site and all its links but also being lost to all those visitors who depend on the site's content and services (Levine 2003).

Obvious as it seems, organizers point out, any online or telephone support network must be tested prior to launching it, to make certain it works properly (Mahoney 2000): with both teleconferencing and online forums, the rule of thumb, unfortunately, is that whatever can go wrong, will! Technology fails—calls disconnect, servers go down. Having a tech-savvy individual available to maintain the system and troubleshoot for problems is essential.

## Marketing

Once a network is operational, it needs to make itself known. The sponsoring organization's staff, many of whom may be caregivers themselves, is the place to start. Mailing flyers or postcards to the organization's database, and news releases or flyers to community newspapers, is also critical to raising awareness of the program. Contacting other organizations with similar client or membership bases is important, too; the organizers of AlzOnline call it "influence the influencers," making those in the eldercare community—area agencies on aging, community-based agencies, senior centers, consumer organizations—aware of their services (Glueckauf and Loomis 2003). Professional conferences are opportunities to disseminate information as well. And narrowly targeted paid advertising may prove affordable and cost-effective.

Technology is making it easier for caregivers to communicate with each other and with professionals through a variety of forums. While there is great promise in these developments, it is also prudent to temper enthusiasm for these advances with recognition of the great diversity of caregivers and their needs, and the difficulty of evaluating the services provided.

This is a movement still in its early stages, one that bears careful nurturing *and* critical monitoring.

## Acknowledgments

Many thanks to all those who provided information on telephone- and Internet-based support programs for caregivers:

Laura J. Bauer, the Rosalynn Carter Institute
Debra Dickerson, North Texas Health Care System/
    VA Hospital-Dallas
Laura Gitlin, Thomas Jefferson University
Myra Glajchen, Beth Israel Medical Center
    Department of Pain Management
Robert L. Glueckauf, University of Florida
Carolyn Johnson, Caregivers in Action
Kathy Kelly, Family Caregiver Alliance
Allen Levine, formerly of CancerCare
Tianna Moscinski, Senior Services of Albany
Fay Radding, formerly of DOROT-USA

## References

Bauer LJ. Personal communication, October 2002.

Brennan PF, JL Overholt, G Casper, and A Calvitti. 1995. Elders using a computer network: Profiles of a champion. *MedInfo* 8(Pt 2): 1545.

Brown R, K Pain, C Berwald, P Hirschi, R Delehanty, and H Miller. 1999. Distance education and caregiver support groups: Comparison of traditional and telephone groups. *Journal of Head Trauma Rehabilitation* 14(3): 257-68.

Colantonio A, C Cohen, and M Pon. 2001. Assessing support needs of caregivers of persons with dementia: Who wants what? *Community Mental Health Journal* 37(3): 231-43.

COR Health LLC. 2001. Online support groups: High on benefits, low on cost. *Internet Healthcare Strategies Newsletter* 3:1-4.

Czaja SJ and MP Rubert. 2002. Telecommunications technology as an aid to family caregivers of persons with dementia. *Psychosomatic Medicine* 64(3): 469-76.

Disease Management Advisor Newsletter. 2000. Online support: Chronically ill patients report benefits, high levels of satisfaction. *Disease Management Advisor* 6(10): 158-61.

Feldman MD. 2000. Munchausen by Internet: Detecting factitious illness and crisis on the Internet. *Southern Medical Journal* 93(7): 669-72.

Fox S and D Fallows. 2003. Internet health resources: Health searches and e-mail have become more commonplace, but there is room for improvement in searches and overall Internet access. Pew Internet & American Life Project. www.pewinternet.org/pdfs/PIP_Health_Report_July_2003.pdf Accessed July 22, 2004.

Gitlin L. Personal communication, October 2002.

Glajchen M. Personal communication, October 2002.

Glueckauf RL and JS Loomis. 2003. Alzheimer's caregiver support online: Lessons learned, initial findings, and future directions. *NeuroRehabilitation* 18(2): 135-46.

Han HR and AE Belcher. 2001. Computer-mediated support group use among parents of children with cancer—an exploratory study. *Computers in Nursing* 19(1): 27-33.

Humphreys K, A Winzelber, and E Klaw. 2002. Psychologists' ethical responsibilities in Internet-based groups: Issues, strategies, and a call for dialogue. *Professional Psychology: Research and Practice* 31(5): 493-6.

Hunt GG. 1998. Technologies to support carers. *Studies in Health Technology and Informatics* 48:158-64.

Klemm P, K Reppert, and L Visich. 1998. A nontraditional cancer support group: The Internet. *Computers in Nursing* 16(1): 31-6.

Levine C. 2003. *Making room for family caregivers: Seven innovative hospital programs.* New York: United Hospital Fund.

Mahoney DMF. 2000. Developing technology applications for intervention research: A case study. *Computers in Nursing* 18(6): 260-4.

Perron B. 2002. Online support for caregivers of people with mental illness. *Psychiatric Rehabilitation Journal* 26(1): 70-7.

Pierce LL, V Steiner, and AL Govoni. 2002. In-home online support for caregivers of survivors of stroke: A feasibility study. *Computers, Informatics, Nursing: CIN* 20(4): 157-64.

Steiner V and LL Pierce. 2002. Building a web of support for caregivers of persons with stroke. *Topics in Stroke Rehabilitation* 9(3): 102-11.

Stewart MJ, G Hart, K Mann, S Jackson, L Langille, and M Reidy. 2001. Telephone support group intervention for persons with hemophilia and HIV/AIDs and family caregivers. *International Journal of Nursing Studies* 38(2): 209-25.

White MH and SM Dorman. 2000. Online support for caregivers: Analysis of an Internet Alzheimer mailgroup. *Computers in Nursing* 18(4): 168-76.

# PART IV

# *Resources*

# 20  On the Quest for Resources: A Guide for Caregivers and Professionals

*Alexis Kuerbis, with Andrea Y. Hart*

Among the difficult, frustrating, and tiresome tasks that caregivers must face, finding information, services, resources, and sources of support for care recipients and themselves is one of the most daunting. I spent close to a year researching this chapter, yet even with the luxury of doing so as part of my full-time job, without the urgency of being a hands-on caregiver, I was frustrated by the results. After spending countless hours on the Internet, sorting through dozens of books, and calling hundreds of organizations, I found that the information I was given was often limited, redundant, or out of date. There is an ocean of information out there, but it is often only an inch deep. While on my quest, however, I began to identify strategies that are likely to make the search faster, easier, and a little less frustrating.

- **Do not hesitate to give this job to someone else.** Friends, family, or even acquaintances will often ask a caregiver if there is anything that they can do to help. Looking for information and resources is an ideal task to pass on to someone else because it consumes excessive amounts of time and energy, two things that are most precious to a caregiver. What's more, the resulting information can be easily conveyed to the caregiver when the work is done. High school or college students in the family may be able to take on this research project.

- **If you can, use the Internet.** The Internet is an easy and quick way to obtain information for caregivers. Whether it is a Web site that specializes in providing moral support, a list of links to Web sites of disease-related organizations, a source of literature about medical conditions, or a means of ordering helpful books or supplies, the Internet offers an easy, convenient, and quick way to begin to find the help you need. If you do not have Internet access from your home, try your local library, schools, hospitals, or other community agencies, which may offer Internet access either for free or for a small fee. The time you spend looking for Internet access will pay off in the hours this helpful technology can save you.

The Web can be particularly useful when looking for books related to caregiving or home care. Even if a caregiver has the time to search in person, it is likely that many of the most helpful books for caregivers will not be on the shelves at local bookstores. A caregiver can order these books over the Web, making the search faster and easier.

One caveat: information on the Internet is variable and sometimes inaccurate. It is important, therefore, not to rely on one site alone. Also, be sure to check out the sponsoring organization. Is it a reputable and reliable source of information? What is its financial stake, if any, in the information provided? When was the Web site last updated? If the site provides medical or scientific information, does it offer citations for the research or information provided?

- **Be sure to use *both* the Internet and the telephone to obtain information.** Just as different agencies sometimes provide conflicting or contradictory information about the same topic, there are often discrepancies between the information an organization posts on its Web site and the information it sends through regular postal mail. That is why it is important to consult and compare all sources of information from an organization. Because the Internet provides an inexpensive and easy way to post a wide range of information, an organization's Web site usually has a more complete description of the types of services it offers than its printed pamphlets. A packet received in the mail is more likely to be tailored to your needs, however. A good practice is to look at an agency's Web site before calling to talk to one of its representatives.

- **Many agencies will send you information that overlaps with or repeats information you have already received from other organizations**. Many organizations refer their callers to the same national or specialized organizations. If you obtain a good list of places to call for help, therefore, do not waste your time looking for other lists until you have exhausted your current one.

- **Before you call an agency, write down specific questions to ask the agency representative, and be as concrete and detailed as possible.** When you call an agency or organization for information, rarely will you get the opportunity to speak with someone—instead of hearing a recording—the first time you call. Even if you do, chances are the person on the other end of the line will give you the most general and brief overview, take down your name and address, and then end the conversation as quickly as possible. That is why you must be prepared. By looking on the Internet first, you can gather enough information to identify specific questions and needs. If you are at the very beginning of your search for resources or have just recently become a caregiver, this may be particularly difficult. Taking time to assess your situation and your concerns, however, will save a lot of time in the long run. Take advantage of the fact that there is actually someone on the line to talk to you. If you find this person helpful, get his or her name and ask to speak with him or her if you need to call again. Many times, even after I asked specific questions, I received only general information that was not helpful, and had to call back to clarify my needs. Knowing who to speak with and what to ask for enabled me to get what I needed much more quickly. Bear in mind that this process can take months, though, so save time by having your questions ready.

- **Expect a delay in receiving information you have requested.** Many organizations have a heavy workload, which delays their sending the information to you right away. Make sure you let the agency know that you need the information as soon as possible, and ask for information over the phone to tide you over until you receive materials in the mail. If you have not received anything within two weeks, chances are you never will. Do not hesitate to call back and request the information again. Usually, a second request receives prompt attention.

- **If you have to leave a message when you phone an organization, be sure to call again.** Many agencies that help caregivers are too small to have someone available to answer the phone more than a few days a week. If this is the case, you will probably reach a voice-mail system or answering machine. Leave a message, but be sure to call again if you have not heard back in a few days. Sometimes it took organizations several weeks to return my call. At times, depending on the agency and the services it provides, it may not be worth the effort to call again. Following up, however, even several times, always produced the best results.

- **Consider major disease-specific organizations for general information.** Some large disease-specific organizations, such as the American Heart Association and the American Cancer Society, have an extensive amount of general information about caregiving and potentially helpful referrals that are useful and relevant to most caregivers, even if their loved one does not suffer from heart disease or cancer. Call and ask for their general information packets—you may find helpful resources in them.

- **Be creative.** Many of the services offered by even the largest agencies do not serve everybody. Even caregivers who live in a large metropolitan area, who are more likely to have resources available to them than those living in rural areas or outside city limits, are often ineligible for services for myriad inconsistent and dumbfounding reasons. It is in just such frustrating circumstances that being creative about finding resources can be the best tactic. That means creating your own personal resource network. This could include contacting community-based agencies to find out what kinds of support services are available in your area. It could involve contacting your local grocery or drugstore to make special arrangements for home delivery of food, medications, or other items. You might consider contacting local businesses, boys and girls clubs, or schools to find out if they have special volunteer programs that might be of assistance. Being creative could also include speaking with government representatives for help, support, and referrals to services. Some places may seem unorthodox but may also be able to provide valuable assistance. It never hurts to ask for what you want; when you do, people can usually find a way to accommodate you and your needs.

- **BE PERSISTENT.** No matter how much you may want to, do not give up. You may have to go through several series of phone calls, letters, agencies, programs, and institutions to get what you need. The saying "the squeaky wheel gets the oil" is unfortunately true. People out there can help you. It just might take a lot of time and energy to get their attention.

What follows is a guide to organizations, Web sites, and books—some well known and some more obscure—that are promising sources of help. Most of the national organizations listed here have state or local chapters; states and larger cities also have departments or offices on aging, chronic care, and related issues, useful for accessing local resources. The few local listings included here also have information useful to a wider audience. Keep in mind that addresses and contact information are likely to change over time, and it is always important to double-check a source's reputation for accuracy. This is not a comprehensive list, but a good place to start.

## Organizations with General Information for Professionals and Caregivers

*American Heart Association*
National Center
7272 Greenville Avenue
Dallas, TX 75231-4596
(800) AHA-USA1 (242-8721) (toll free)
Women's Health: (888) MY-HEART
  (694-3278) (toll free)
www.americanheart.org

*American Stroke Association*
(AHA-affiliated organization;
  use AHA address)
(888) 4-STROKE (478-7653) (toll free)
www.strokeassociation.org

*Centers for Medicare and Medicaid Services (CMS)*
Information Clearinghouse
7500 Security Boulevard
Baltimore, MD 21244-1850
(877) 267-2323 (toll free)
(410) 786-3000
Medicare Hotline: (800) MEDICARE
  (633-4227) (toll free)
TTY: (866) 226-1819 (toll free)
  *or* (410) 786-0727
www.cms.hhs.gov
  or www.medicare.gov

*Family Caregiver Alliance*
690 Market Street, Suite 600
San Francisco, CA 94104
(800) 445-8106 (toll free)
(415) 434-3388
www.caregiver.org

*Friend's Health Connection*
PO Box 114
New Brunswick, NJ 08903
(800) 48FRIEND (483-7436) (toll free)
(732) 418-1811
www.48friend.org

*Hospice Association of America (HAA)*
228 7th Street, SE
Washington, DC 20003
(202) 546-4759
www.hospice-america.org

*Lighthouse International*
111 East 59th Street
New York, NY 10022-1202
(800) 829-0500 (toll free)
(212) 821-9200
TTY: (212) 821-9713
www.lighthouse.org

*National Alliance for Caregiving*
4720 Montgomery Lane, 5th Floor
Bethesda, MD 20814
(301) 718-8444
www.caregiving.org

*National Family Caregivers Association*
10400 Connecticut Avenue, Suite 500
Kensington, MD 20895-3944
(800) 896-3650 (toll free)
(301) 942-6430
www.nfcacares.org

*National Hospice and Palliative
Care Organization*
1700 Diagonal Road, Suite 625
Alexandria, VA 22314
(703) 837-1500
Helpline: (800) 658-8898
www.nhpco.org

*Rosalynn Carter Institute for
Human Development*
800 Wheatley Street
Americus, GA 31709
(229) 928-1234
www.rci.gsw.edu

*Well Spouse Foundation*
63 West Main Street, Suite H
Freehold, NJ 07728
(800) 838-0879 (toll free)
(732) 577-8899
www.wellspouse.org

*YAI/National Institute
for People with Disabilities*
460 West 34th Street
New York, NY 10001-2382
(212) 273-6182
www.yai.org

## Travel Planning

*HouseCalls USA*
470 Biltmore Way
Coral Gables, FL 33134
(877) 24HRDOC (244-7362) (toll free)
www.hoteldocs.com
- Arranges 24-hour medical,
  dental, and optical services
  for individual travelers, as well
  as telephone consultations
  with medical personnel

*Mobility International*
PO Box 10767
Eugene, OR 97440
(541) 343-1284
www.miusa.org
- Provides advice and technical
  assistance to educational institutions
  on how to include people with
  disabilities in exchange programs

*New Directions*
5276 Hollister Avenue, Suite 207
Santa Barbara, CA 93111
(888) 967-2841 (toll free)
(805) 967-2841
www.newdirectionstravel.com
- Sponsors annual travel
  programs throughout the U.S.
  and abroad for people with
  developmental disabilities

## Aging and Eldercare Service Organizations

*American Association of Homes and Services for the Aging*
2519 Connecticut Avenue, NW
Washington, DC 20008-1520
Community Assistance Information:
    (800) 677-1116 (toll free)
(202) 783-2242
www.aahsa.org

*AARP (formerly American Association of Retired Persons)*
601 E Street, NW
Washington, DC 20049
(800) 424-3410 (toll free)
www.aarp.org (English and Spanish)

*Eldercare Locator Service*
(800) 677-1116 (toll free)
TDD/TTY: (202) 855-1234
www.eldercare.gov

*Friends and Relatives of Institutionalized Aged*
11 John Street, Suite 601
New York, NY 10038
Helpline: (212) 732-4455
www.fria.org

*Medicare Rights Center*
1460 Broadway, 17th Floor
New York, NY 10036
(212) 869-3850
HMO Hotline: (800) HMO-9050
    (466-9050) (toll free)
www.medicarerights.org

*National Association of Area Agencies on Aging*
927 15th Street, NW, 6th Floor
Washington, DC 20005
(202) 296-8130
Area Agency Offices: (800)
    677-1116 (toll free)
www.n4a.org

*National Association of Professional Geriatric Care Managers*
1604 North Country Club Road
Tucson, AZ 85716-3102
(520) 881-8008
www.caremanager.org

*National Center on Elder Abuse*
1201 15th Street, NW, Suite 350
Washington, DC 20005-2842
(202) 898-2586
www.elderabusecenter.org

*National Institute on Aging*
Public Information Office
Building 31, Room 5C27
31 Center Drive, MSC 2292
Bethesda, MD 20892
(301) 496-1752
www.nih.gov/nia (English and Spanish)

## Disease-Related Organizations

AIDS
*Gay Men's Health Crisis (GMHC)*
119 West 24th Street
New York, NY 10011
(800) AIDS-NYC (243-7692) (toll free)
Hotline: (212) 807-6655
www.gmhc.org

*National AIDS Hotline*
*Centers for Disease Control*
*and Prevention*
(800) 342-AIDS (342-2437) (toll free)
Spanish: (800) 344-SIDA (344-
    7432) (toll free)
TTY: (800) AIDS-889
    (243-7889) (toll free)
www.ashastd.org/nah

*National Association*
*of People with AIDS*
1413 K Street, NW, Suite 700
Washington, DC 20005
(202) 898-0414
www.napwa.org

Alzheimer's Disease
*Alzheimer's Association*
225 North Michigan Avenue, Suite 1700
Chicago, IL 60601-7633
(800) 272-3900 (toll free)
(312) 335-8700 (direct line)
www.alz.org

*Alzheimer's Disease Education*
*and Referral Center (ADEAR)*
PO Box 8250
Silver Spring, MD 20907-8250
(800) 438-4380 (toll free)
www.alzheimers.org

Cancer
*American Cancer Society (ACS)*
1599 Clifton Road, NE
Atlanta, GA 30329
(800) ACS-2345 (227-2345) (toll free)
www.cancer.org (English and Spanish)

*Cancer Care, Inc.*
275 Seventh Avenue
New York, NY 10001
(800) 813-HOPE (813-4673) (toll free)
(212) 712-8080
www.cancercare.org

*National Cancer Institute—*
*Cancer Information Service*
NCI Public Inquiries Office, Suite 3036A
6116 Executive Boulevard, MSC8322
Bethesda, MD 20892-8322
(800) 4-CANCER (422-6237)
    (toll free—English and Spanish)
TTY: (800) 332-8615
cis.nci.nih.gov/

Others
*American Diabetes Association (ADA)*
Attn: National Call Center
1701 North Beauregard Street
Alexandria, VA 22311
(800) 342-2383 (toll free)
www.diabetes.org

*American Parkinson Disease Association*
1250 Hylan Boulevard, Suite 4B
Staten Island, NY 10305
(800) 223-2732 (toll free)
www.apdaparkinson.org

*Amyotrophic Lateral*
*Sclerosis Association*
27001 Agoura Road, Suite 150
Calabasas Hills, CA 91301-5104
Information and Referral: (800)
    782-4747 (toll free)
(818) 880-9007
www.alsa.org

*Brain Injury Association.*
8201 Greensboro Drive, Suite 611
McLean, VA 22102
(800) 444-6443 (toll free)
(703) 761-0750
www.biausa.org (English and Spanish)

*Lupus Foundation of America*
2000 L Street, NW, Suite 710
Washington, DC 20036
(800) 558-0121(toll free)
(800) 558-0231 (toll free, Spanish)
(202) 349-1155
www.lupus.org

*NAMI—National Alliance*
*for the Mentally Ill*
Colonial Place Three
2107 Wilson Boulevard, Suite 300
Arlington, VA 22201-3042
HelpLine: (800) 950-NAMI
    (950-6264) (toll free)
(703) 524-7600
TDD: (703) 516-7227
www.nami.org

*National Institute of Arthritis*
*and Musculoskeletal and*
*Skin Diseases (NIAMS)*
Information Clearinghouse
National Institutes of Health
1 AMS Circle
Bethesda, MD 20892-3675
(877) 22NIAMS (226-4267) (toll free)
(301) 495-4484
TTY: (301) 565-2966
www.niams.nih.gov

*National Institute of Neurological*
*Disorders and Stroke*
PO Box 5801
Bethesda, MD 20824
(800) 352-9424 (toll free)
(301) 496-5751
TTY: (301) 468-5981
www.ninds.nih.gov

*National Multiple Sclerosis Society*
733 Third Avenue
New York, NY 10017
(800) FIGHTMS (344-4867) (toll free)
www.nmss.org

*National Organization*
*for Rare Disorders*
55 Kenosia Avenue
PO Box 1968
Danbury, CT 06813-1968
(800) 999-6673 (toll free)
(203) 744-0100
TDD: (203) 797-9590
www.rarediseases.org

## Places to Visit on the World Wide Web

Useful as the Internet is, bear in mind that Web addresses may change and sites may be taken out of service. If you are having trouble accessing one of the sites listed here, try double-checking the address by using a Web search engine or phoning the sponsoring organization. Some sites are clearly commercial, but offer useful information along with the products or services they may be marketing.

*AEGIS HIV/AIDS*    www.aegis.com
- This massive Web site connects thousands of bulletin boards from around the world to pool information and resources for those who are infected or are caring for someone who is infected with HIV. This is an excellent place to start a resource search. It lists many links, articles, fact sheets, question-and-answer sessions, sources of emotional support, and other resources, and provides information to help users understand the disease, treatment options, and secondary illnesses.

*Aging with Dignity*    www.agingwithdignity.org
- This not-for-profit organization's Web site features a downloadable form for a living will, called Five Wishes, that covers medical, emotional, and spiritual needs.

*Alzheimer's Caregiver Support Online*    www.AlzOnline.net
- This Web site—a collaboration of the State of Florida Department of Elder Affairs, the University of Florida, and the University's Center on Telehealth and Healthcare Communications—provides professionally moderated telephone and Web-based education and support for caregivers of persons with progressive dementia. Caregivers can also use the site to access a resource center and health professionals.

*American Health Assistance Foundation (AHAF)*    www.ahaf.org
- This Web site describes AHAF's research and education programs on age-related and degenerative diseases, and its emergency financial assistance for eligible families with a loved one suffering from Alzheimer's. The site also has an "ask the expert" section for caregivers with general questions about Alzheimer's.

*American Health Care Association (AHCA)*    www.ahca.org
- AHCA is a national federation of long-term care providers and state health organizations. Its Web site can connect individuals with their state agencies, for information about state health care policies and services.

*America's Health Insurance Plans*   www.ahip.org
- This site offers good consumer information and has brochures and online order forms for other publications.

*Association of Cancer Online Resources*   www.acor.org
- This site offers a number of online support communities for cancer patients and their families.

*Beth Israel Hospital's Department of Pain Medicine and Palliative Care*
www.stoppain.org
- The New York–based hospital's Department of Pain Medicine operates professionally moderated teleconferences and Webcasts for caregivers of medically ill persons around the country; it also offers access to local and national resources, an online newsletter, and a resource directory. [Tel.: (212) 844-1713]

*The Body*   www.thebody.com
- For persons with or affected by HIV/AIDS, this comprehensive site provides information and resources, including a bulletin board through which individuals can communicate directly and an "ask the experts" link to health professionals.

*CancerCare*   www.cancercare.org
- This organization's Web site provides information and support programs for persons caring for cancer patients. It operates support groups via a closed bulletin board facilitated by oncology social workers. A prerequisite for participation is the patient's being in or recently completing treatment; CancerCare also requests a three-month commitment, although groups may run as long as six months, depending on caregiver needs. Participation is free and confidential.

*Caregiver-Information.com*   www.caregiver-information.com
- This site offers basic, practical information for people caring for loved ones with Alzheimer's disease, stroke, or brain injury. Information is well organized and presented in lay terms—describing the three conditions in detail, discussing current treatments, and offering tips to make life easier while caregiving.

*Caregivers.com*   www.caregivers.com
- This information and referral network for caregivers and seniors is most notable for its selection of search engines on housing, geriatricians, lawyers, care managers, and hospice care.

*Caregiver Survival Resources*   www.caregiver.com
- This Web site has all types of resources and a wealth of information, both general and specific. There are links to other health-related Web sites, information on books, and disease-specific resources.

*Caregiving Online: Wellness for Caregivers of an Aging Relative, Friend or Neighbor*
www.caregiving.com
• An offshoot of *Caregiving* newsletter, this Web site offers emotional and social support from fellow caregivers via support groups, message boards, and links to other resources. Users can register for e-groups tailored to their length and level of caregiving and relationship to the care recipient. The site also provides useful information on how to access community resources.

*ElderWeb*   www.elderWeb.com
• This site features articles and links on finance and law, housing and care, long-term care insurance, organizations, and events, with a display adaptable for accessibility.

*Family Caregiver Alliance*   www.caregiver.org
• Although the organization itself serves only clients in California, its Web site offers helpful information and resources for both in- and out-of-state caregivers of persons with brain injury, dementia, Huntington's disease, or Parkinson's disease. Caregivers can access experts, online forums, and a library.

*Fodor's Travel Online Resource Center*   www.fodors.com/traveltips/disabilities
• Although not geared specifically to caregivers or care recipients, this travel Web site does have a section offering useful information, resources, and travel tips for those with special needs while on vacation.

*GetCare.com*   getcare.com
• Offering information on long-term care choices, this site helps users decide what options are best for them and their loved ones. There is an online needs assessment, a description of six basic forms of long-term care services, and a search engine to locate providers nationwide.

*Health Finder, by the U.S. Department of Health and Human Services*
www.healthfinder.gov
• This federally funded search engine can help users find links to all types of health information, in both English and Spanish.

*HealthWorld Online*   www.healthy.net
• This site caters mainly to persons interested in homeopathy, holistic health, and other forms of alternative medicine, but also offers general health information, including medical articles and links to related Web sites.

*The Healthy Caregiver*   www.healthycaregiver.com
• This online magazine for caregivers is another good place to begin seeking caregiver resources. It has an "ask the expert" section, and links to other caregiver organizations, disease-related organizations, and government agencies.

*Little Brothers—Friends of the Elderly*  www.littlebrothers.org
- This national not-for-profit organization is committed to relieving the isolation and loneliness of the elderly.

*Medicare Information*  www.medicare.gov
- This is the official U.S. government site for Medicare information.

*Mr. Long-Term Care*  www.mr-longtermcare.com
- This commercial site claims to be the most comprehensive resource on long-term care on the Internet, with information about resources and advocacy, columns by long-term care experts, news, interviews, and extensive links.

*National Alliance for the Mentally Ill (NAMI)*  www.nami.org
- NAMI's Web site has a range of resources for persons suffering from mental illness, their families and caregivers, and professionals, including books and articles, support groups, and general information. The organization also offers a Family-to-Family Education Program, a free course that teaches families about treatment options for and coping with illnesses such as schizophrenia, bipolar disorder (manic depression), clinical depression, panic disorder, and obsessive-compulsive disorder.

*National Association for Home Care and Hospice*  www.nahc.org
- This association provides an online guide on how to choose a home care agency, and lists resources by state.

*National Consumers League*  www.natlconsumersleague.org
- Dedicated to protecting consumer interests, this site teaches consumers how to guard against fraud and how to report it, and offers information on dangers of over-the-counter drugs. It also represents consumers on marketplace and workplace issues.

*The National Council on the Aging*  www.ncoa.org
- The Web site of this agency, which works with the elderly to achieve optimum health, independence, and financial security, offers health insurance counseling, related links, resource information, and software.

*National Organization for Empowering Caregivers (NOFEC)*
www.nofec.org *or* www.care-givers.com
- An affiliate of "Empowering Caregivers," a Web site started by a caregiver, NOFEC's Web site also provides a forum for caregivers to interact with one another, and offers numerous online resources and an "ask the experts" link.

*National Spinal Cord Injury Association*    www.spinalcord.org
- This is an interactive Web site for people with spinal cord injuries. It has a comprehensive collection of fact sheets, book lists, and other information, and a directory of local chapters.

*Nolo.Com, Inc.: Law for All*    www.nolo.com
- This Web site offers articles, books, and other information on topics ranging from how to deal with employment issues to wills and power of attorney.

*OncoLink, University of Pennsylvania Cancer Center*    www.oncolink.upenn.edu
- With extensive information and statistics for patients with all types of cancer and their caregivers, this Web site features an "ask the expert" section, information on disease management, a clinical trial matching and referral service, and disease-specific e-mail support groups.

*Ourelders.org*    www.ourelders.org
- Developed to provide comprehensive links to Web sites with information and resources for the elderly, this site is particularly helpful in its numerous links to Alzheimer's disease–related sites.

*Project Inform*    www.ProjectInform.org
- Another great place to start a search for resources on HIV/AIDS, this Web site has a wealth of information and links on new treatments, and offers assistance to the newly diagnosed with understanding the disease and choosing appropriate therapy. Text is available in both English and Spanish.

*Resources for Enhancing Alzheimer's Caregiver Health (REACH) Project*
www.edc.gsph.pitt.edu/reach
- The National Institute on Aging and the National Institute of Nursing Research are currently funding caregiver interventions at six universities around the U.S.; information on the program is available at this Pittsburgh-based site.

*The Spinal Cord Injury Ring—Resources for the Disabled*
www.makoa.org/sci.htm
- This site offers a broad range of resources for spinal cord injury, including numerous links, and interactive forums including a bulletin board, chat rooms, and a listserv where caregivers can log on to exchange information or obtain support.

*The TBI Help Desk for Caregivers*    www.tbihelp.org
- Although locally sponsored by New York's Jamaica Hospital Medical Center, and no longer offering updated interactive features, the Help Desk offers enough archived information and links to caregiving resources to remain useful to a broad audience of caregivers of persons suffering from traumatic brain injury.

*Worldwide Congress on Pain, Dannemiller Memorial Educational Foundation*
www.pain.com
- Geared to both consumers and professionals, this site offers news, interactive question-and-answer sessions, access to doctors for questions regarding pain management, interviews, and a list of local pain clinics.

## Selected Books for Professionals and Caregivers

Many of the wide variety of books on family caregiving are available in libraries or can be purchased in bookstores or online. For titles that may be harder to find, ordering information is included.

Berman, Claire, and Brody, Deborah, eds. *Caring for Yourself While Caring for Your Aging Parents: How to Help, How to Survive.* New York: Henry Holt, 2001 (revised).

*Fodor's Great American Vacation for Travelers with Disabilities*, 2nd edition. Westminster, MD: Random House, 1996.

Ilardo, Joseph, and Rothman, Carole R. *I'll Take Care of You: A Practical Guide for Family Caregivers.* Oakland, CA: New Harbinger Publications, 1999.

Lustbader, Wendy, and Hooyman, Nancy R. *Taking Care of Aging Family Members. A Practical Guide.* New York: Free Press, 1994.

Mace, Nancy L., and Rabins, Peter V., MD, MPH. *The 36-Hour Day: A Family Guide to Caring for Persons with Alzheimer's Disease, Related Dementing Illnesses, and Memory Loss Later in Life*, 3rd edition. Baltimore: Johns Hopkins University Press, 1999.

McFarlane, Rodger, and Bashe, Philip. *The Complete Bedside Companion.* New York: Simon and Schuster, 1998.

McLeod, Beth W. *Caregiving: The Spiritual Journey of Love, Loss, and Renewal.* New York: John Wiley and Sons, 1999.

Meyer, Maria M., with Derr, Paula, RN. *The Comfort of Home: An Illustrated Step-by-Step Guide for Caregivers*, 2nd edition. Portland, OR: CareTrust Publications, LLC, 2002.

Mintz, Suzanne Geffen. *Love, Honor, and Value: A Family Caregiver Speaks Out about the Choices and Challenges of Caregiving.* Sterling, VA: Capital Books, 2002.

Mittelman, Mary S., and Epstein, Cynthia. *The Alzheimer's Health Care Handbook: How to Get the Best Medical Care for Your Relative with Alzheimer's Disease, In and Out of the Hospital.* New York: Marlowe, 2003.

Morris, Virginia, and Butler, Robert. *How to Care for Aging Parents: A Complete Guide.* New York: Workman, 1996.

Richards, Marty, ed. *Eldercare: The Best Resources to Help You Help Your Aging Relatives.* Issaquah, WA: Resource Pathways, 2000. [To order: (888) 702-8882.]

Strong, Maggie. *Mainstay: For the Well Spouse of the Chronically Ill*, 3rd edition. Northampton, MA: Bradford Books, 1997.

Susik, D. Helen. *Hiring Home Caregivers: The Family Guide to In-Home Eldercare*. San Luis Obispo, CA: American Source Books, 1995.

Visiting Nurse Associations of America. *Caregiver's Handbook: A Complete Guide to Home Health Care*. New York: DK Publishing, 1998.

Wilkinson, James A. *A Family Caregiver's Guide to Planning and Decision Making for the Elderly*. Minneapolis: Fairview Press, 1999.

# Contributors

**Terry Altilio**, MSW, ACSW, is coordinator of social work for the Department of Pain Medicine and Palliative Care at Beth Israel Medical Center in New York City. She is secretary of the New York State Cancer and AIDS Pain Initiative, on the advisory board of the American Alliance of Cancer Pain Initiatives, and chair of the Pain and Palliative Care Special Interest Group of the Association of Oncology Social Workers, as well as a lecturer in the Schools of Social Work of both New York University and Smith College. Ms. Altilio is a recipient of a Social Work Leadership Award from the Open Society Institute's Project on Death in America.

**Jane Bendetson**, MFA, MA, is a freelance writer living and working in Maine, an emeritus adjunct professor, and a former teacher in the independent schools of New York City. She has been the recipient of grants from the National Endowment for the Humanities and the National Endowment for the Arts. A speaker on aphasia at conferences on stroke, she is co-facilitator of the Portland Aphasia Support Group of the New England Rehabilitation Hospital, Portland, ME, and facilitator of a caregiver support group.

**Jeremy Boal**, MD, is the director of the Visiting Doctors Program of the Mount Sinai Medical Center in New York City. He graduated from the Medical College of Wisconsin and completed an internal medicine residency and geriatrics fellowship at Mount Sinai, where he is currently an assistant professor of medicine and geriatrics, as well as a faculty member of the Hertzberg Palliative Care Institute. His principal interests include home care, professionalism in medical education, ethics, and palliative care in the home.

**Kathryn Cooper Corley**, MS, is the busy mother of three young children, ages 3 to 11. Additionally, she provides contract services for the Tennessee Early Intervention System, conducting developmental assessments and consulting with families. She volunteers as parent coordinator for T.C. Thompson's Children's Hospital Project DOCC program and has participated as a panelist or panel moderator for Project DOCC in Memphis, Chicago, and Atlanta. She is a member of the United Mitochondrial Disease Foundation.

**Lynn Friss Feinberg** is deputy director of the National Center on Caregiving at the San Francisco–based Family Caregiver Alliance, which works nationally to advance the development of high-quality, cost-effective policies and programs for caregivers. She currently directs a 50-state survey, funded by the U.S. Administration on Aging, to profile the state of the states in family caregiver support, and is the co-principal investigator of a research study on decision making and service use in caregiving families. A member of the board of directors of the American Society on Aging, an associate editor of the *Journal of Mental Health and Aging*, and a member of the American Society on Aging's *Generations* editorial board, Ms. Feinberg holds a master's degree in social welfare and gerontology from the University of California at Berkeley.

**Gladys González-Ramos**, PhD, MSW, is associate professor at the New York University School of Social Work, and adjunct associate professor of neurology at the NYU School of Medicine. She has more than 25 years of experience in the field of mental health, particularly in delivery of services to Hispanic families. In collaboration with the director of field services of the National Parkinson Foundation, Inc., she has been developing educational and outreach programs for underserved populations affected by Parkinson's disease. In addition, Dr. González-Ramos maintains a private practice in New York City.

**Andrea Y. Hart** is a program associate in the United Hospital Fund's Division of Education and Program Initiatives. She is responsible for coordinating research and programmatic activities for the Families and Health Care Project and the Medicine as a Profession Forum, a collaboration of the Fund and the Open Society Institute.

**Gail Gibson Hunt** is president and CEO of the National Alliance for Caregiving, a nonprofit coalition of nearly 40 organizations focused on support for family caregivers and the professionals who work with them. The Alliance conducts research and policy analysis, develops programs for family caregivers, and works to increase public awareness of caregiving issues. Ms. Hunt headed her own aging services consulting firm for 14 years, and was senior manager in charge of human services for the Washington, DC, office of KPMG Peat Marwick.

**Barry J. Jacobs**, PsyD, a clinical psychologist and family therapist, is director of behavioral sciences for the Crozer-Keystone Family Practice Residency in Springfield, PA. He is also an adjunct faculty member of the Institute for Graduate Clinical Psychology of Widener University, the University of Pennsylvania School of Nursing, and the Temple University School of Medicine. He has made presentations and served as a consultant for the Rosalynn Carter Institute for Human Development, the Well Spouse Foundation, the National Family Caregivers Association, and the United Hospital Fund. His book on families and illness is forthcoming from Guilford Publications.

**Robert L. Kane**, MD, is professor and Minnesota Chair in Long-Term Care and Aging, Division of Health Services Research and Policy, at the University of Minnesota School of Public Health, Minneapolis. His research and extensive writings have focused on both the outcomes of clinical care and organization of care, with special attention to the chronic-care needs of older adults.

**Shoshanna Korn-Meyer**, CSW, has been a social worker in the Mount Sinai Medical Center Visiting Doctors Program since August 2001. She received a master's degree in social work from Columbia University in 1997.

**Alexis Kuerbis**, CSW, is project director of the onsite CASAWORKS for Families research project of the National Center on Addiction and Substance Abuse at Columbia University, at the Mount Sinai Medical Center Alcohol and Other Drug Treatment Program, where she also provides individual, group, and family addiction treatment. Ms. Kuerbis teaches courses on alcoholism and on bioethical issues at St. Joseph's College of New York in Brooklyn. Formerly, she was the program associate at the United Hospital Fund's Families and Health Care Project.

**Carol Levine** joined the United Hospital Fund in 1996 as director of its Families and Health Care Project. She continues to direct the Orphan Project: Families and Children in the HIV Epidemic, which she founded in 1991. She was director of the Citizens Commission on AIDS in New York City from 1987 to 1991. As a senior staff associate of the Hastings Center, she edited the *Hastings Center Report*. In 1993 she was awarded a MacArthur Foundation Fellowship for her work in AIDS policy and ethics.

**Jeffrey Nichols**, MD, is the chief of geriatrics at Cabrini Medical Center in New York City. He is also the medical director of the Cabrini Center for Nursing and Rehabilitation, senior medical director for Saint Cabrini Nursing Home in Dobbs Ferry, NY, and assistant medical director for geriatrics and palliative care of the Cabrini Hospice. Dr. Nichols serves on advisory committees of the national Alzheimer's Association and its New York City chapter, and on the faculty of both the Mount Sinai School of Medicine and Weill Cornell Medical College. A graduate of Columbia College and Cornell University Medical College, Dr. Nichols is board certified in internal medicine, geriatrics, and hospice and palliative care.

**Raymond L. Rigoglioso** is a freelance writer and editor.

**Timothy J. Sweeney** is the senior program officer for the Diversity and Inclusiveness Program at the Evelyn and Walter Haas, Jr., Fund, a family foundation based in San Francisco. Previously, he served as deputy executive director of the Empire State Pride Agenda, a New York State gay and lesbian advocacy organization. From 1990 to 1993 he was executive director of Gay Men's Health Crisis, the nation's oldest and largest AIDS service, education, and advocacy organization.

**Lili Toborg**, GNP/ANP, has been with the Mount Sinai Medical Center Visiting Doctors Program since 2000. She received a BA from Hampshire College and a BS and Masters of Nursing Science degrees from Columbia University.

**Donna L. Wagner**, PhD, is director of gerontology and director of the Center for Productive Aging at Towson (MD) University; she is also a professor in the College of Liberal Arts there, and chair of the Interdisciplinary Council. Prior to coming to Towson she was the vice president for research and development of the National Council on the Aging in

Washington, DC. A fellow of the Gerontological Society of America and active member of the Association for Gerontology in Higher Education, Dr. Wagner is also a correspondent for the UK Third Age Employment Network, chair of the Maryland Consortium of Gerontology in Higher Education, and a consultant for the National Alliance for Caregiving and Family Caregiver Alliance.

**Joan C. West** taught elementary school for more than 30 years and was a master teacher, mentor, and staff developer. She is currently an adjunct instructor at St. Joseph's College in Patchogue, NY, where she supervises student teachers in their field placements and teaches education/child study courses. Joan also makes student presentations and runs staff development and parenting workshops for CAPS (Child Abuse Prevention Services) on Long Island.

**Rabbi Gerald I. Wolpe**, MA, MHL, DD, is rabbi emeritus of Har Zion Temple, Penn Valley, PA, where he served as senior rabbi for 30 years, until retiring in 1999. He is the director of the Jewish Theological Seminary's Louis Finkelstein Institute of Social and Religious Studies, and a senior fellow of the University of Pennsylvania's Center for Bioethics. He is also a member of the Aphasia Society of America's board of directors, and of the National Institutes of Health Commission on Genetics and the Community.

**Carol Ann Young**, MA, is an elementary school teacher in New York City; she has served as a New York City Teaching Fellow and member of AmeriCorps. Previously, she was a graphic designer for 30 years in the field of advertising and promotion. She is a member of the Board of Overseers of the Brookdale Center on Aging of Hunter College and was a member of the Mount Sinai Hospital's Caregivers and Professionals Partnership Program's steering committee.

**Connie Zuckerman**, JD, is an attorney and bioethics consultant. Her areas of expertise include geriatric patient care and palliative care. Ms. Zuckerman has held positions as associate director of the Center for Ethics in Medicine at Beth Israel Medical Center in New York, and as project director of the Hospital Palliative Care Initiative at the United Hospital Fund.

# Index